The Street Clinic

The Street Clinic

10 Young Lives on the Frontline of Gang Culture

Dorcas Gwata

PICADOR

First published 2026 by Picador
an imprint of Pan Macmillan
The Smithson, 6 Briset Street, London ECIM 5NR
EU representative: Macmillan Publishers Ireland Ltd, 1st Floor,
The Liffey Trust Centre, 117–126 Sheriff Street Upper,
Dublin 1 D01 YC43
Associated companies throughout the world

ISBN 978-1-0350-0691-5

Copyright © Dorcas Gwata 2026

Photographs © Chanel Pinnock 2026

The right of Dorcas Gwata to be identified as the
author of this work has been asserted in accordance with
the Copyright, Designs and Patents Act 1988.

All rights reserved. No part of this publication may be reproduced,
stored in a retrieval system, or transmitted, in any form, or by any means
(including, without limitation, electronic, mechanical, photocopying, recording
or otherwise) without the prior written permission of the publisher.

Pan Macmillan does not have any control over, or any responsibility for,
any author or third-party websites (including, without limitation, URLs,
emails and QR codes) referred to in or on this book.

1 3 5 7 9 8 6 4 2

A CIP catalogue record for this book is available from the British Library.

Typeset by Clare Sivell
Printed and bound in the UK using 100% Renewable Electricity by CPI Group (UK) Ltd

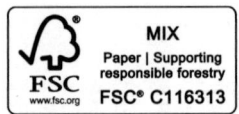

This book is sold subject to the condition that it shall not, by way of
trade or otherwise, be lent, hired out, or otherwise circulated without
the publisher's prior consent in any form of binding or cover other than
that in which it is published and without a similar condition including this
condition being imposed on the subsequent purchaser. The publisher does not
authorize the use or reproduction of any part of this book in any manner
for the purpose of training artificial intelligence technologies or systems.
The publisher expressly reserves this book from the Text and Data Mining
exception in accordance with Article 4(3) of the European Union
Digital Single Market Directive 2019/790.

Visit **www.picador.com** to read more about
all our books and to buy them.

To my son, Chakanyuka. With every word of this book,
I thought of you, your safety and your tomorrow.
Thank you for the beautiful light you bring into my world.

Contents

A Note on the Text	ix
Introduction: The Nurse	1
1. Fuz: The Courtroom	7
2. Abdul: The Estate	29
3. Lori: The Cafe	58
4. Amir: The Mosque	84
5. Jordan: The Church	115
6. Jevaun: The Football Pitch	143
7. Louise: The City	171
8. Hanad: The A & E Department	196
9. Zane: The House	224
10. Alex: The School	255
Acknowledgements	286
Notes	289
A Note on the Photography	293
About the Author	294

A Note on the Text

To respect the privacy of clients, friends and colleagues, I have altered a great many details. All the stories of clients I have worked with are composite. To maintain patient confidentiality, I have anonymized names and changed demographic information, clinical details, dates, times and places.

Confidentiality in nursing practice is sacred and grounded in both ethics and law. As a nurse I recognize the vulnerabilities of young people I have looked after and care deeply about all the patients that I have worked with throughout my career. For this reason I have gone to immense lengths to protect their confidentiality and ensure that this book is morally binding and also abides by the law. The photographs by Chanel Pinnock do not depict the places or people in the stories that follow.

Introduction: The Nurse

'One in five NHS staff in the UK report a non-British nationality. Yet their global expertise, cultural insights and leadership skills are often overlooked.'

THIS BOOK TELLS the stories of ten lives, based on real events and experiences but sufficiently altered to protect identities and maintain privacy. It tells how people in search of safety and stability in our British cities – whether they are British citizens who have been born and raised here, or people like me who have uprooted their lives to be here – can too often become victims of violence and also perpetrators of violence.

I want these stories to speak to misconceptions of youth violence and vulnerability and to reveal how fear produces the wrong government policies. I want to showcase the defiance of women of colour who are protecting their sons and daughters as best as they can in the face of systems that do not always work for them. I want to dig into our understanding of the faith, sexuality and morality of our immigrant communities. I want to investigate how dark stigma and suicide can tear families and communities apart, and how the unspoken culture of honour killings lingers for some of our young British women. And, along the way, I share my own story of being an immigrant who started at the bottom of the heap, as a cleaner in a hospital in Edinburgh, and had to climb over what felt like barbed wire to get on in the NHS. Through it all, we get a bird's-eye view of the true colours of London society: how the institutions that are put in place to protect us can also contribute to the destruction of our lives.

Already an experienced clinical nurse specialist with established global-health experience, in 2013 I was asked to fill a role created by the office of the then mayor of London, Boris Johnson. My role would explore the mental-health needs of young people and their families affected by gang culture: knife crime, sexual exploitation and human or drug trafficking. The Children's Society estimates that as many as 46,000 children in England are involved in gangs, with 4,000 of those in London alone. Many of the young people I worked with had been excluded from mainstream education, some had learning difficulties, and most were from minority backgrounds, with all the social and economic constraints which that often entails. London is a particularly multicultural city; many of my patients are of African, Caribbean or Middle Eastern descent, second- or third-generation immigrants whose parents or grandparents came to London in search of safety, only to lose their lives – sometimes literally – to gang violence.

Somewhat counterintuitively, by extrapolating research lessons from low-income countries, I was able to apply them to our high-income country. Employing all my skills – from the HIV/AIDS programmes I'd worked on in Zimbabwe to the UK and West African diaspora programmes I'd supported during the Ebola pandemic – I rolled up my sleeves and started to tackle the mental-health aftermath of the then undeclared epidemic of knife crime in young Black and ethnic-minority groups in London. Working in a team dedicated to saving young people's lives, I was the immigrant nurse who went where most healthcare professionals would not dare to tread. And my clinic became known as the Street Clinic.

The Street Clinic seeks to explain why young men who have been stabbed on the streets of London, where I nursed, continue to recycle violence. It explores their vulnerability and how their trauma is never really addressed because our mental-health services are not designed with them in mind. My own experiences of racism and exclusion have brought me closer to the experiences that my patients face. When my younger brother was stabbed in London, my own world was turned upside down: he

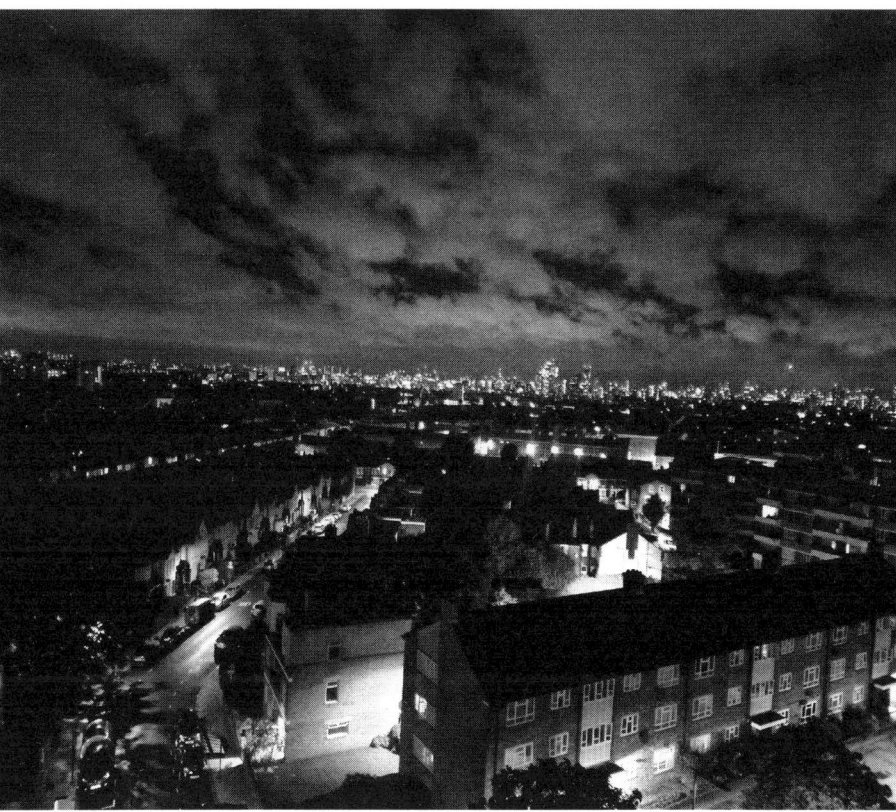

lives with his injuries; his trauma is our collective trauma. I am not just an occasional visitor to the communities I serve; I am a part of that community.

The stories contained in these pages include that of Fuz, who has learning difficulties, has long been excluded from mainstream education and lives in poverty in one of London's most expensive postcodes. He had been involved in petty crime, which slowly escalated to robberies of iPhones and expensive bikes, but then the violence took the darkest possible turn. I write about attending Fuz's trial at the Old Bailey. There is Amir, a teenage boy involved in a fatal fight outside his school gates on the last day of term. I spent the afternoon with his mother and sister in the women's quarter at a mosque. In Hanad's story, we hear how he was brought into A & E, depressed and distressed, by his sister and mother. His cousin had committed suicide and Hanad, unwilling to show his vulnerability, had no idea how to cope with the situation and his emotions. With his mental health compromised, he too was now at risk. I nursed Hanad at his most vulnerable moment and helped him to decide his future. And then there is Lori, who suffered a sexual assault that made her turn to cannabis and to consider self-harm. Her mother was just fifteen when she fell pregnant with Lori and, having always struggled to support her, she found it difficult to meet Lori's needs. But, despite of all this trauma, Lori responded well to therapy with me and has recovered.

Over ten chapters, *The Street Clinic* looks at how I have cared for each young person, while painting a bigger picture of the societal issues we face here in Britain, where the rate of knife crime continues to grow. I want to share these stories of vulnerability and strength because they're important. They reveal the lives of young people we may not always come across – and, if we do, we might not truly see them. My writing honours the might of the NHS and sheds light on the everyday experiences of minority groups both accessing and delivering its services. Where I have castigated the system, it is because I adore it and want it to work for all our communities. Mostly, I am simply in awe of the resilience of the young people I have been lucky enough to serve. Their engagement and desire for a safer London pushed my clinical skills and led me to bring innovation to the role. I salute the people who work on the frontline of our NHS and the multi-agencies that work alongside our healthcare system, tirelessly and often invisibly. This book honours their enormous contribution to the NHS.

Dorcas Gwata

1. Fuz: The Courtroom

'At least one in three people moving through the justice system are thought to be neurodivergent.'

It is a warm, late summer morning, and as I carefully navigate my way through the crowds of people gathered in the foyer of the Old Bailey, I notice how each person sags like a worn-out mattress, ground down by the austere surroundings and wearied by the frantic comings and goings of which they, reluctantly, are a part. Huddled closely together, each small group's conspiratorial whispers are barely audible beyond the inner sanctum they've created with their hunched bodies. This is both a grand public space and an intensely private space. I adjust my unravelling headwrap, its incongruous bright colours reflecting prettily in the tiles that line the otherwise muted corridors, and edge my way into the observation gallery of Court Six.

People slowly take their seats, the wooden gallery benches groaning with age, defying the strict court rules that demand silence. The low hum of shifting, unsettled bodies in the almost reverential surroundings feels offensive, too loud, and I ease myself down with care. Beside me, a plump, middle-aged woman of Arab appearance sits anxiously rocking forwards and backwards, and the bench creaks painfully with her every move

– a sympathetic acknowledgement of the collective pain that's already palpable, or perhaps a cry of protest at our collective weight. She too looks worn out. Her prayer beads are just visible beneath the voluminous sleeves of her elaborate dress and she is worrying them through her fingers. What brings her here? I wonder. Is she a relative of the victim, perhaps? I am equally nervous, but I know that I will find community in our shared vulnerability.

The Old Bailey sits at the heart of London's legal district, a stone's throw from the majestic St Paul's Cathedral, where glamorous royal weddings have dazzled the world, and close to Fleet Street, where news personnel and journalists, for over four hundred years, created and crafted stories to feed a news-hungry market. The Central Criminal Court of England and Wales – where major criminal cases are heard, most of which involve serious assault and, often, murder – has long borne witness to evidence that is hard to hear and often bitterly contested. Criminal gangs have been tried here for heinous offences that have both defiled and defined our society.

Gang demographics will vary depending on the time and place. The make-up of the gangs appearing at the Old Bailey have evolved over the years. One might be deceived into thinking that London's violence is synonymous with minority groups, but this is not the case. In the late 1960s, the East End-born Kray brothers met their fate here at the Old Bailey, their signature style of violence particular to their generation and, even now, unmatched in its fearsomeness. Yet, for all the differences, I can't help but think that the trial unfolding here today, which is also founded in gang activity, has its parallels.

The mood at the Old Bailey is rarely one of celebration, and today is no exception. A great deal of psychological trauma resides in the court's footprint and it's impossible not to be sensitive to its history. It's a troubled place, where criminal meets

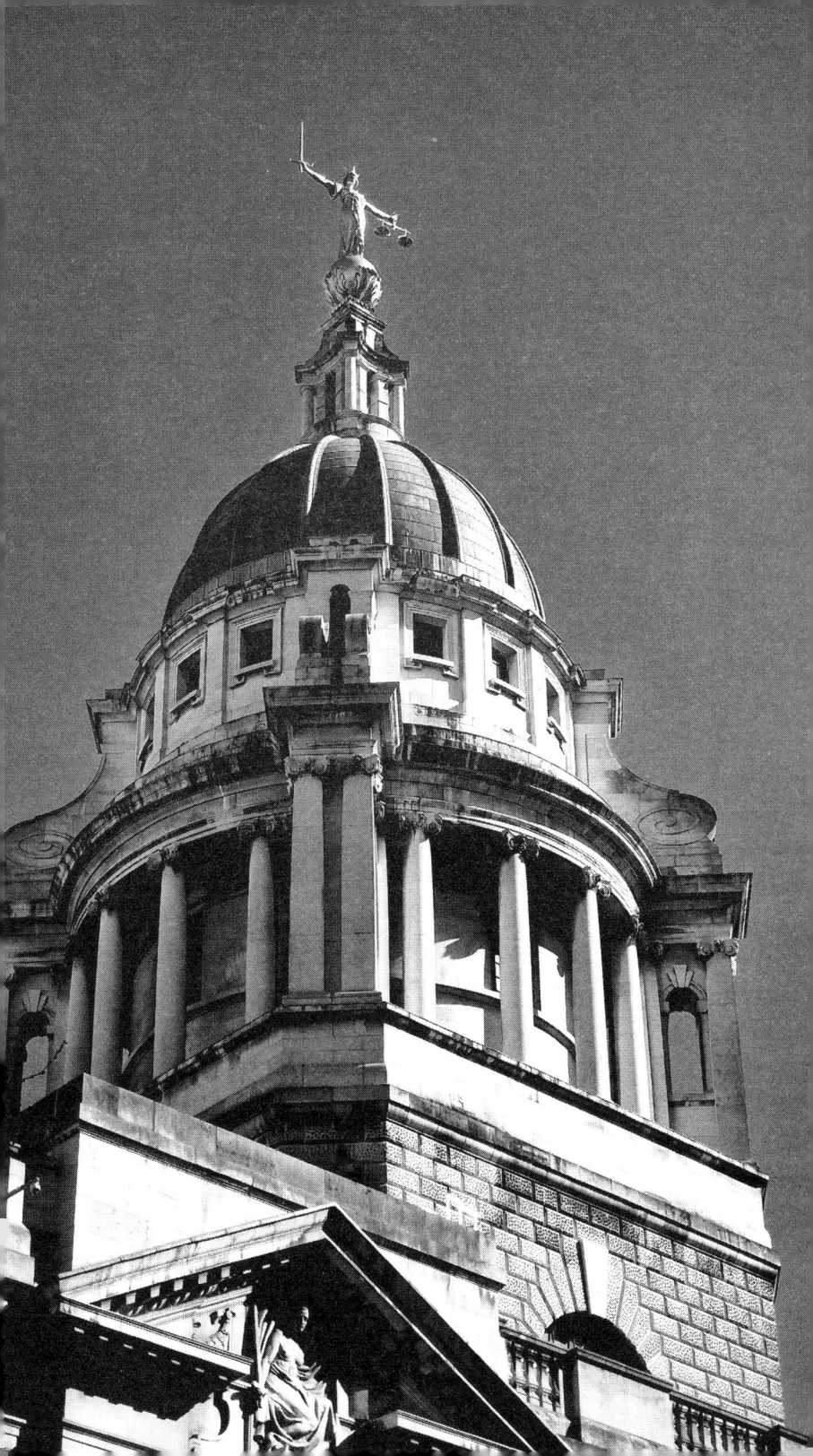

victim once more, or perhaps comes face to face with the family and friends the victim has left behind. To muddy the waters, the accused have invariably been victims of crime themselves. In my experience as a nurse, I have seen how those accused of the crime of stabbing another person have often been the victim of several stabbings in the past. It can be a vicious cycle. And it's why I am here today – to be in the presence of one of my young clients who is accused of a crime that very nearly killed a stranger on a London street. I want to be here partly to find closure in a case that has troubled me, but also to try to understand how the intersectional issues of gangs, mental health and justice operate. There is almost nothing in my nursing training that has prepared me for this moment. These are uncharted waters for most of us in nursing and I am having to dig deep to find my composure as I search for answers that I may never find.

We are all here for different reasons. I know that, of those seated around me, some are here to see justice carried through with all the blunt force of the law. They want to look the perpetrators in the eye and see them suffer, as they are suffering. They want the punishment to be protracted and painful. But, whatever the verdict, there are no winners here. Both the victims and the criminals have already lost in life in some fundamental way.

Standing up a little for a better view, my eyes scan the room for the accused, darting across unfamiliar faces of all ages, and eventually come to rest on three young men, two of whom are of mixed heritage and one white Caucasian. They are sitting with their heads tilted to one side or the other as though they're listening out for something. Their youthful bodies are draped in casual suits, a dress code that's a world away from their usual attire of hoodies and trainers. Their typical street clothes convey a sense of territory, identity, power and dominance, the very characteristics that define gangs. Today, however, they need to project a different message. They are in another's space now. They are humbled, fully aware that they have no power here. Their futures are in someone else's hands.

These three young men have been accused of carrying out a string of street robberies, snatching handbags and iPhones, on a night that ended with one person being stabbed – a stranger to them all, left with life-changing injuries. So violent was the attack that he very nearly lost his life. The victim, a twenty-one-year-old British man of Turkish descent, had been studying engineering at a local university. He had no criminal record and no affiliations with the accused. He was standing outside a coffee shop, smoking a cigarette and making a call, when the expensive and clearly covetable iPhone X Max was snatched from his hand from behind. He gave chase and a fight broke out, according to the police report. A single stab wound ruptured his shoulder, and another pierced his lower abdomen. He was rushed to the local trauma centre, where he was treated and hospitalized.

A London crime scene like this will invariably invite crowds to gather. Local residents and shopkeepers, astonished that the city's bloody underbelly has found its way to their doorstep – *Doesn't this sort of thing always happen to someone else?* – huddle together in collective grief. Scores of young people wearing hoodies and drop-down pants will slowly circle the area, like wary hyenas. In fight-or-flight mode, they never linger, scattering the moment the police sirens become audible in the distance. Some communities will take solace from speaking highly of the victim, if it's someone known to them. *He was a good boy. He always helped his mother with the shopping. He comes from a nice family.* But even they are cautious of being caught up in the ensuing investigations and will hurry back to their homes and watch proceedings unfold from behind net curtains. They know that gang members are merciless to witnesses, and some have paid the ultimate price for speaking out. In the aftermath of an incident like this, fear hangs in the air. But it is fused with defiance and a determination to carry on, despite the violence and the horror. And, for most people, life does carry on.

Looking around the courtroom as it continues to fill up, half out of my seat, my eyes keep coming back to Fuz, who was nicknamed by the gang members for his learning difficulties. Of the three young men on trial today, I know him best. Like most people, I know him by this street name, and the name being used in the courtroom makes it feel as though we're talking about a different person. Fuz, I've learned, has a strong desire to please his 'elders' – gang members who dominate the drug scene across London's council estates. He is seventeen, but with the mental age of a fourteen-year-old. Fuz cannot read much. He is highly impulsive. He has had poor school attendance since the early years of secondary education. As I watch him, I wonder whether he has the capacity to fully grasp the weight of today's proceedings. For me, while I know the law must take its course, I dread the outcome.

Fuz is accused of buying the knife that stabbed the victim that night. His co-defendants are both accused of actual bodily harm, which is a lighter charge than attempted murder. Fuz also wielded the knife at some point – or, at least, that is the accusation being made by the prosecution. All three are accused of robbery. These three young street warriors, as vulnerable as they are powerful and bound so tightly by blood, crime and violence, are now divided in the courtroom, each pointing the finger at the others. A so-called cut-throat trial. Though seated together, the reality is that each man stands alone, accountable for his own actions. Each is desperate to save his own skin.

Fuz had been referred to my clinic through the Gangs Unit. His keyworker Aaron was clear when he made the referral that

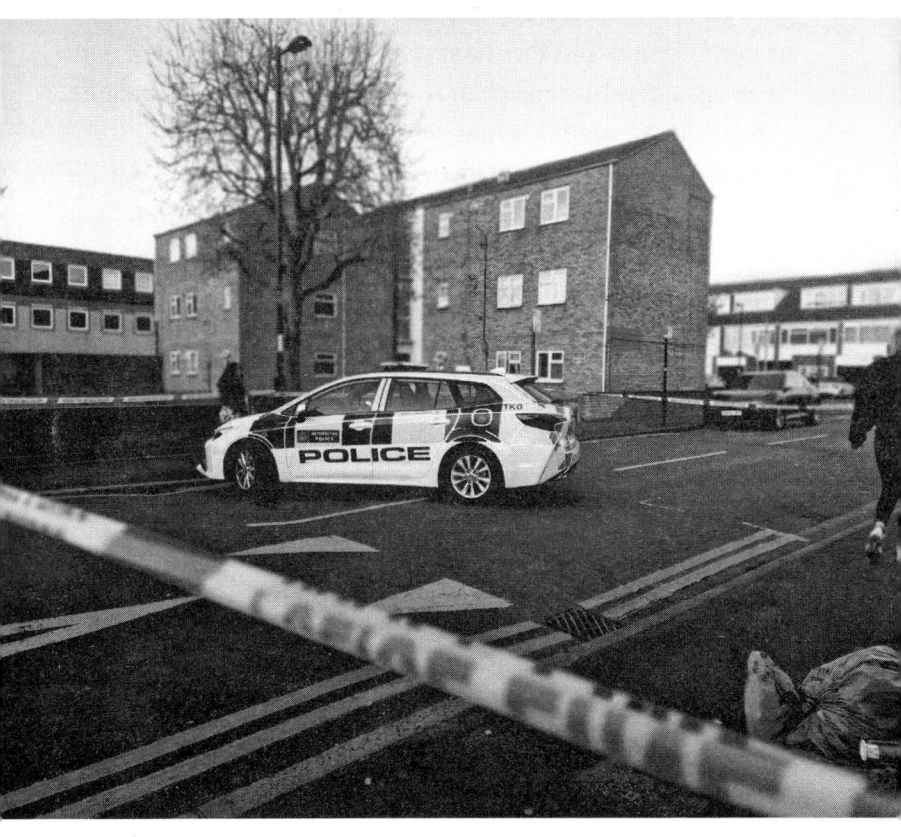

Fuz was a 'follower', a people pleaser; with his limited cognitive abilities, Fuz was happy to obey instructions given by those whom he admired, invariably older gang members. It is not fathomable that he bought the knife of his own volition. His learning difficulties are precisely why he is such an asset to gang members, and a liability to himself. And now he is here, sitting on a wooden bench in the Old Bailey, accused of a serious crime that has already changed an innocent's life for ever and will now change his. I hope that Fuz, whose life has been so unfair, will be tried justly by a jury of his peers. I pray that their findings will be fair to Fuz and to the victim too.

More people take their places on the bench, and I shuffle along to accommodate them before realizing I have no further space to move into. I perch precariously on the edge, and the bench groans again. The woman with the beads is praying in whispers, which fly urgently from her pursed lips. I edge forward, straining to look out over the rows of seating. I wish Fuz could see me. I'd like to make eye contact with him, to let him know I am here for him. I know he will be terrified. I know he needs my support.

Fuz has grown up in care, moving from care home to care home throughout his childhood. He was moved from one borough to another in his early teens, stepping into new territory at a difficult age. He struggled to make sense of his new environment, which had long been volatile with youth violence. He quickly became low-hanging fruit for the entrenched drug dealers lurking in the neighbourhood. Unable to secure his own safety, he looked to these elders for it and they duly provided a sense of family. It's a curious kind of belonging that is only understood by those who belong. These seasoned drug dealers prey on vulnerable and fragile young people, who most likely come from broken homes and challenging backgrounds. The council estates are usually their recruiting ground. They understand poverty well, and are likely to have lived through it themselves. They know how stressed parents are about the bills that need to be paid. They know that adolescents who come from fractured or toxic homes often don't have much of what they desire, so they recruit them onto the streets in a process that's innovative and creative. And the lost adolescent is oblivious to how they're being groomed.

First, there is the offer of food: a free burger and chips, perhaps, which fills the hunger void that has long been a part of their home life. A free pair of expensive trainers and an iPhone turn up from nowhere and are gratefully received. Then, a switch-up: they're asked to move a package from A to B. Perhaps, as a reward, there's the offer to pay off some of their mother's bills, which will help to ease her stress. She too is now trapped in the game. And the game, which plays out in the streets, defines who is safe and who is not, who is protected by the influential kingpins and who is not. Following a structure that's strictly hierarchical, recruits rise through the ranks, commanding more respect as they do so. It's the powerful gang leaders at the top of the food chain who tend to survive; they're rarely ever caught with the stash because that's someone else's job. Someone like Fuz, who was a seasoned 'runner' for these bigger boys – the young men who have done their time and now control street activities from behind the scenes.

Safety and perceptions of safety have a whole different meaning for young people like Fuz who are caught up in petty crime and violence. Safety isn't a protective parent or an adult guardian looking out for you, a schoolteacher or a sports coach. It's defined by the street you can or cannot cross, and the shopping mall you can treat like home, or need to avoid. For young people like Fuz, hanging out in Oxford Street – while the tourists and shoppers obliviously hustle and bustle around them – may well mean carrying a knife for protection. Fuz knew the street codes by the time he was thirteen years old. His father is doing time for murder and his mother has served a short prison sentence for possession of drugs with intent to supply. The odds have always been against him.

*

As Fuz got older, the streets became bloodier. Across the UK, youth violence and knife stabbings peaked in 2017, claiming 285 lives that year, with some victims as young as thirteen. The number of young people living with the after-effects of injury and trauma increased significantly between 2017 and 2018, and London was not the only city in the UK grappling with an epidemic of knife crime. In Scotland, Glasgow was facing its own challenges, wrapped in layers of social inequality that had mounted up over the years. There, huge numbers of predominantly young white men were losing their lives in violent incidents. The city responded by successfully rolling out a public-health framework to tackle knife crime, with commendable results. The number of people murdered or living with the effects of knife crime began to reduce, and with this evidence there was pressure on London to roll out a similar public-health framework to protect its most vulnerable, many of whom were living in our Black communities.

Fuz is a part of that London community. He is Black. He has learning difficulties. He is unquestionably vulnerable. With his complex needs, he was a time bomb, but unfortunately it remains the case that there are few services available to support young people like him. Our NHS mental-health services were not designed with people like Fuz in mind, people whose chaotic and unstructured lives mean they're unlikely to attend an NHS or social-services appointment. They quickly find their way onto the *did not attend* checklist that will exclude them from further offers of help. It's a system that does little to try to understand the context in which these vulnerable youths live, and to work around them and with them. The recognition that more needed to be done to support young people like Fuz led to the creation of a London Gangs Unit – a multi-agency team, drawing on specialisms from across health and social care – and my role within it. I began working with some of the finest professionals, whose commitment to saving young people's lives is as strategically informed as it is compassionate.

Nurses who specialize in learning difficulties usually work within the confines of a clinic or a large hospital, or a health facility for outpatients who attend sessions regularly or irregularly, depending on need. Some may do community visits. However, these will be specifically commissioned and they are not necessarily inclusive of those most in need of them. My clinic is different. When I started my specialist clinical nursing role within the Gangs Unit, it was the only nursing role in the country specializing in gangs and mental health. And, while services are still developing, it's not enough to capture the vast number of children living with neurodivergent needs who are on the cusp of criminality and whose safety is highly compromised due to gang association.

The strength and success of the London Gangs Unit has been defined by its ability to access young people in the most creative and innovative ways. It's a team of people who understand young people's challenges, who know that many young people who are caught up in gangs don't get out of bed until midday, which means interventions are designed around their lifestyle. The team understands that, despite criminality, young people and their families are often true to their culture and faith, so they seek to access them in these spaces – whether that's McDonald's or Starbucks, a barber shop or a church or mosque – immersing themselves within the communities they seek to support. It is a street clinic which speaks to the needs of young people like Fuz.

My clinics shift; they are not static. They are highly mobile and adaptive, like the cleaning trolley I pushed in my first job with the NHS. It means I go where I'm needed. This often includes prisons. I may spend several days visiting young people in Belmarsh Prison in south-east London, and then move on to delivering mental-health workshops in Brixton and Feltham prisons. Invariably, the young prisoners I work with are from minority groups. Some have converted to Christianity, Buddhism or Islam while inside, and some will come out of their incarceration rehabilitated. But others are hardened by the experience, and getting through to them is difficult. We do all we can while these young men are with us and we have access to them, but mental healthcare for young offenders leaving prison is still fragmented and poor. The risk of reoffending or reverting to gang culture is high. In the absence of sustainable, meaningful support, these young men return to what they're familiar with, often at high cost.

The art of nursing requires that we view our patients in the most human terms, including those who have committed crimes. Indeed, many of my general nursing colleagues are used to treating patients who might have been injured whilst carrying out heinous acts. Some will later be held in institutions such as Broadmoor Hospital, but they are our patients through and through. My adolescent patients, who potentially carry knives, who pose a huge risk to themselves and others, are equally capable of committing horrific crimes. But as a nurse I am able to see beyond the violence and danger that someone like Fuz represents to the public. Instead, I could immediately see that Fuz was a petrified six-foot-tall adolescent who had learned to mask his fears with cannabis and an overconfident street bravado, which he was delighted to find attracted as many girls as enemies. There was something that connected me to Fuz, a therapeutic bond built on trust, compassion and care, which quickly came to the surface during our time together.

But I always knew his prognosis was poor. In his deepest moments of reflection, when he allowed himself to open up, he shared with me his fears of being stabbed. He knew he was at risk not only from those who openly opposed him – his known enemies – but from the people he called friends, people he hung out with, who were supposed to have his back. These street friendships are built on a tribal allegiance, but they are fragile, volatile. They can't be depended on. They can flip in an instant from camaraderie to chaos, over the loss of some drugs or over a girl – for girls are so often just another possession, something to own, to have control over, to use, something these young men don't want to lose.

As I look down at Fuz from the gallery of Court Six, I understand that he has experienced so much in his short life and that he has learned a lot. But he has many blind spots and he failed to see the enemies emerging from within his group of friends. His learning difficulties make him incapable of assessing risk, unable to pause and think through the consequences of his behaviour. Fuz's world is no bigger than the postcode he inhabits, a piece of London that is insignificant in size, yet means everything to him. Fuz is facing the possibility of a long prison sentence and I am wondering how he will cope with this.

While a lot of work and money goes into keeping young people out of prison, the numbers who nonetheless end up there remain unacceptably high, with Black adolescents disproportionately represented, certainly in England. Many from minority groups continue to slip through the net, sometimes with catastrophic results. Prison can either make them or, more often, break them. It is a test of survival for these young people and, while rehabilitation programmes are available and can be effective, they are often poorly accessed. Even when the government throws money at the problem, it is not clear how best to spend that money: to those involved, the roots of the problem are often obscure. The hoped-for solution turns out to be too little, and too late. Then, with a change of leadership comes new ideas, new policies. But these policies continue to miss the mark. And as the debate about what to do rages on, the young people keep suffering. Fuz had been at risk for a long time. We should not only have seen this latest crisis coming, but we should have had the measures in place to prevent it.

What I'd been able to do in my work with him was also too little, and too late.

*

I first met Fuz at a youth club. I was running a workshop on mental health and cannabis use. The room was filled with young people at risk and the youth workers who were concerned about their mental well-being. In the workshop, drawing on recent research, I made the link between cannabis and common mental-health disorders such as anxiety and depression, the clinical components which can lead to fear, violence and isolation in young people. As a way to engage the young people in the room, I diluted my language, referring to mental-health issues as 'problems' and 'stress' and 'headaches', rather than the loaded and stigmatized medical diagnoses that can make people nervous and defensive. I was very intentionally general in the way I referred to trauma and fear – these were not young people who wanted to be told they were scared. Fuz was in the audience. He had recently been stabbed and, while he'd recovered physically, his youth workers had noticed that he'd become angrier and more explosive. They were worried that he had started to carry a knife for protection, and that, rather than making him safer, it merely exposed him to even greater danger. Given his inherent vulnerability, as well as his poor emotional regulation, the youth workers' team had referred him for mental-health work because they felt he was at risk.

My clinic is different from the generic office-based clinic that is widely available to young people with mental-health challenges. Mine has to be adaptive to the environment that young people move in. While the interventions are often the same, the delivery is innovative. I have had to adjust my working practice considerably. In an office setting, I would get adolescents to fill in questionnaires to quiz them about their mental health, gently probing them to try to assess their issues and working out how I could help them. Now, on the streets and in the youth clubs, I do much the same, but without the paperwork; the questions I need answers to are instead filed in my head. Most of my adolescents have poor literacy skills and are unable to read, having left school too soon or having had such poor attendance that they simply never learned.

Interventions with adolescents who have been stabbed, I quickly learned, can be challenging. They are traumatized and even less trusting than before the incident. Beyond the hospital environment, where they have no choice but to seek help for physical injuries, they are reluctant to engage with social services. It takes persistence and a great deal of creative thought to get them on side. But it is possible to turn it around, to pull them out of the cycle of violence and into employment or higher education. When I first met Fuz, I hoped that my clinical expertise would help him to address some of the trauma that had surfaced and which was threatening to sink him.

After the workshop wrapped up, I approached Fuz, who was amusing himself bouncing a basketball in a corner of the hall. He turned and looked at me warily. I knew he was trying to work out if he could trust me. I locked eyes with him and smiled, letting him know again that I was a nurse and that I had a lot of experience looking after young people who were troubled.

It wasn't usual for a nurse to be hanging around with young people in a youth club, he pointed out.

I couldn't pretend that it was. 'No, it's a new idea,' I said. 'But here I am.'

He smiled back and said, 'The last time I saw a nurse was when I was in hospital. I got stabbed, innit.'

There is nothing normal about an adolescent being stabbed. I didn't want Fuz to think for a minute that I might diminish his experiences. On the contrary, I wanted him to know that I cared deeply about him.

'I'm interested in how you're feeling about all that,' I said gently.

I knew better than to ask who had stabbed him, and why, and how it had happened. It wasn't my place, or my job. My concern was with his mental health and well-being.

He bounced the ball a little harder. Anxiety, perhaps. He wasn't used to sharing his feelings. Besides, I knew that there were girls waiting for him outside. I knew that he had to leave, that this wasn't the right time for us to talk.

*

It is hard to comprehend the poverty that exists in Westminster. When you see it, it is an ugly and surprising picture of brutal deprivation, alive and well in the centre of one of the wealthiest cities in the world. Victorian social housing and more modern concrete estates, which sprang up post-war to replace bomb-damaged terraces, are uncomfortably sandwiched between affluent stucco-fronted Victorian villas. The estates have become littered with gangs that control the area, and the primary currency is drugs. Just over the river from the borough of Westminster, in south London, the rave clubs in Vauxhall are a big market for those drugs, and the fight for territory and dominance sometimes spills across the river and back to Pimlico. For many who live there, it's a silent war, a battle that's invisible to those who go about their polite daily business. For people like Fuz, it's a part of life and can't be ignored.

However different the lives of the affluent middle classes are from the lives of young people like Fuz, drugs provide a common denominator. We are a nation deeply immersed in drug use and abuse. Our drugs of choice include heroine and crack cocaine, crystal meth and dexies, and over-the-counter drugs that linger in the body and sometimes produce psychologically bizarre behaviours that surface in our hospitals' accident and emergency departments. During my working life as a hospital cleaner and into the early years of the twenty-first century, when I qualified as a nurse, alcohol abuse and dependency seemed to be the foundation of our social fabric. Now, we are treating drug-abuse cases alongside alcohol abuse, and sometimes the violence that is associated with it. Our national focus on drugs is heavily skewed towards the poorer users – some who are as young as thirteen and are highly exposed to drug use through the adults around them. This focus is important and we should never tire until every child is safe. However, the lack of focus on the middle-class buyers also plays on my mind. Every time an affluent young man or woman working on the trading floor of a City bank, say, or the production floor of a TV company buys cocaine from a seventeen-year-old on a street corner, they too are part of the chain of violence and the trauma that is associated with it.

*

For my first appointment with Fuz, I perched on the edge of a wall near Pimlico Tube station and waited. He had been clear that, while he was happy to meet with me, he could not – or would not – make morning sessions. OK, I'd said. This was nothing new, with my clients; I wasn't going to argue with him. Despite all the things that set me apart from other mental-health professionals, all the lived experience and specialist training which I am able to bring to the table, I knew that it would still take a while to gain Fuz's trust. At the heart of engagement with young people exposed to gang culture is the ability of health professionals to adjust to their lifestyles. And so I sat on the wall and waited.

I needed to catch him in the brief window between his waking up in his own good time and the point in the afternoon when he would disappear into his world of friends, girls, cannabis and whatever dramas the combination of all three would inevitably throw up. But I could see I wasn't the only person waiting for him. A few metres along the wall, one of the girls from the youth club was reapplying her make-up, adding last-minute touches to the already beautiful tones of her delicate brown skin. Glancing up from her mirror, her eyes briefly met mine and her expression confirmed that I had competition for Fuz's time. My window of opportunity had just become a little narrower, but I reasoned that any moment we have to engage with young people is a teachable moment. I had learned to be effective in my communication and interventions, even in a five-minute encounter.

When we both next looked up from our phones, we saw Fuz heading in our direction. It was half past three in the afternoon and he was half an hour late, but it was obvious that he had just woken up. He went to the girl first and they hugged, lightly, in case the streets were watching. This is the time the streets come alive. Fuz stepped away from her and came to settle on the wall beside me. Despite the pressure around him, despite the eyes, Fuz was choosing to engage with my street clinic. Although I would never show it, I was delighted.

The National Institute of Health and Care Excellence (NICE) provides evidence-based recommendations on the best standards of care for the health and social care sector, and it's this standard to which doctors and nurses align our interventions. As nurses, we lean on NICE guidelines to provide the best patient care and improve outcomes. Interestingly, the guidelines specify that adolescents should be offered appointments where they feel most comfortable. I keep this in mind, providing options for meeting places and times. For the young people I work with,

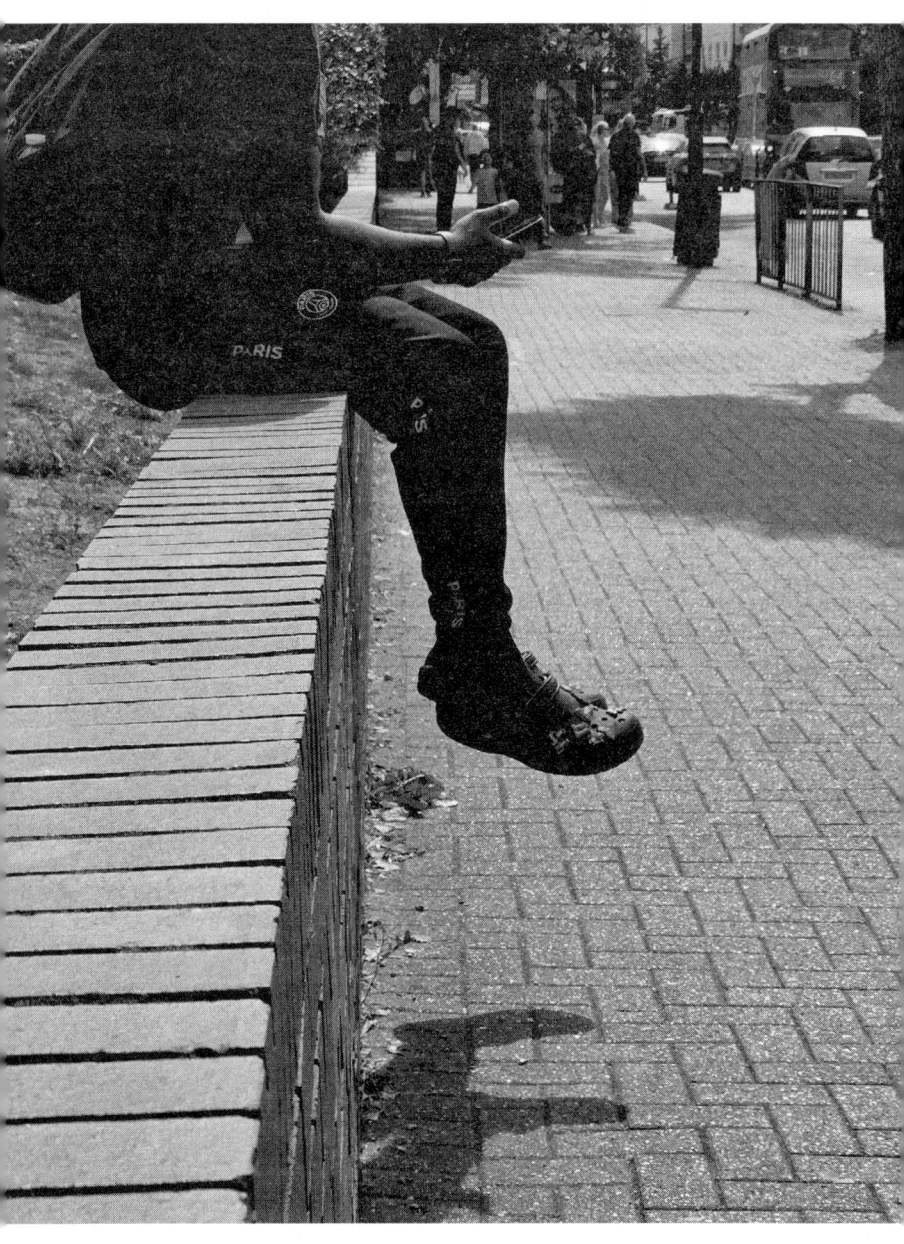

the choice is often determined by safety and time. Had I asked Fuz to meet on the other side of the borough at ten o'clock in the morning, he might not have kept our appointment because he would not have felt safe in another postcode. And he most certainly wouldn't have been awake at that time of the morning.

As I settled into a brief session with Fuz, I thought through the measurement tools that I would usually use in a clinical environment, working out how to apply them to my interaction with him. Concerned about the effect of the stabbing on his sense of safety and mental well-being, I knew that the 'Impact of Events' questionnaire would be best suited to help us explore this. It's a clinical tool used to tease out the extent to which clients have been affected by an incident that may have caused trauma or had a significant impact on their lives. I also had the 'Revised Child Anxiety and Depression Scale' at my disposal – a forty-seven-item questionnaire designed to assess key features of depression and anxiety. I knew it was inconceivable for me to cover everything with Fuz in this one meeting, so I plucked from them the specific questions that would give me an indication of his clinical picture.

But, as always, I began by checking in with him – a simple 'How are you doing?' registering my care and empathy.

'I am alright you know, I am alright,' he answered, looking down at his feet, a standard answer that all my clients tend to give.

Using physical health as an entry point to his mental health, I asked Fuz in a hushed tone about his sleep. In an equally hushed tone, he told me that, despite lying in bed for most of the day, he wasn't really sleeping, that his mind was wandering, reliving the moment when he was stabbed and thinking about how he could have died. I mentally flicked through the trauma-based questions that would allow Fuz to open up about his fear, and he told me that his mind was constantly racing, and that's why he had started smoking cannabis, to calm it down.

Now, to add to it all, Fuz was worried that he'd had a falling-out with one of his best friends. Based on what he knew of the streets, he realized that even a small conflict could turn into a storm, which could leave someone seriously hurt. Or worse. Like so many of the adolescents that I work with, he wasn't equipped with the conflict-resolution mechanisms or emotional regulations required to de-escalate the situation.

He let me know that the stitches from his stab wound had fallen out naturally. I told him that, if he had any concerns, he should see his GP. And, although he said he would, I knew he wouldn't. Fuz, and young people like him, are more likely to come to the attention of the medical services via accident and emergency, via surgical teams and sporadic mental-health interventions than they are via their local doctors' practice. It's only when things have hit rock bottom that they'll seek any kind of help – and, even then, they're likely to discharge themselves against medical and nursing advice, and not show for follow-up outpatient appointments.

It was a complicated situation. But Fuz was talking to me, and that could only be a good thing.

*

In Court Six at the Old Bailey, my hands are sweaty and I am tired. My headwrap is loosening again and I have long lost any sensation in my left leg from perching awkwardly at the end of the bench. We all rise as the judge enters, and the lawyers, administrators, guards and jury eventually retake their seats. As we prepare for the verdict, I can feel the courtroom tensions rise and a profound hush descends. When Fuz is sentenced to prison for many years, I hear muffled wails and the soft sounds of sobbing from around the room. I digest the information in silence. The lady with the prayer beads doubles down on her efforts, her invocations that much louder now. I hope she has included Fuz in her prayers.

There is much debate about whether children should be imprisoned or not, particularly children with mental-health challenges who are predisposed to trauma by virtue of environment or upbringing. Children like Fuz. The intersectionality of social inequality, violent crimes, culture and exploitation provide context that we should fold into these debates; but, for the victims of crime, this context offers no comfort. I understand that and I empathize. The law is rigid, and must do what it must do. I acknowledge that, while I'm able to view Fuz through the deeply compassionate lens nursing requires, others may not have the same capacity. Others, especially the victim's family, will see Fuz only as an attacker who could have murdered someone. As a criminal. To them, he is nothing more than the perpetrator of violence, the instigator of the most painful episode of their lives.

But Fuz is a product of our society. He is ours. He and others like him are a part of us, their actions the result of having followed a particularly difficult pathway through British life. They form a small but significant section of our community that falls through the safety net – a net which is pretty robust, for we have made it as strong as we can. But it's not strong enough to catch the likes of Fuz. Our society has rejected Fuz. Most people turn the other way when they see him – or others like him – coming. Yet these young people live with us and among us. They define who we are.

2. Abdul: The Estate

'Embarrassing or incriminating social media content can become "online collateral" for "hostage taking" that can be used to bind people to the gang, or sanction, coerce, and control them.'

ALL FOUR OF US are huddled around the computer screen, pressed shoulder to shoulder, waiting impatiently to see the photos of eighteen-year-old Abdul. The office air is stale, but outside the November rains are gathering momentum, the steady drumming of the downpour the only sound in the otherwise hushed room. We have just come out of a safeguarding and intelligence meeting, a hub in which healthcare and social-services professionals pool their thoughts, and Abdul's is the case that I have been asked to follow up on.

It's Calvin, one of the youth workers, who has his laptop open, but it's taking an age for him to log in and download the images. We wait, not entirely patiently. Jaden, one of the ex-offenders who has become a youth worker since leaving prison, is hovering over the laptop expectantly. He's six feet tall and his body demands space. While some people might find him threatening – and he will have dominated some territory or other back in the day and instilled fear in fellow gang members and enemies alike – I know him only as docile and caring. I've never asked what the crime was that led to his prison sentence; I want and need to know him only as he is now, not as he used to be. Then there's Mayse, who is specifically commissioned to work with young girls who are exposed to gangs and are vulnerable to exploitation. Always dressed in signature black, she has real presence. She grew up in care; she knows well the issues that our young people are facing. Finally, there is Monty, another youth worker who has come through the youth justice system himself and isn't fazed by much. As things on this case develop, I'm particularly keen to know his views.

All we know at this point is that a few photos of Abdul have been posted online, and in them he is dressed in pink shorts and a white shirt. The word on the street, the urban community which Abdul calls home, is that he is gay. And, for Abdul, that's a problem. He has suffered endless abuse as the pictures have been passed around various social-media platforms with humiliating captions attached. Pink has become the colour of his torment, with girls stopping him in the street to offer him pink scarves or pink socks to shame him. The word spread like a wildfire among the Iranian-British community in the borough, where it's not the norm to see someone of Abdul's ethnic background freely expressing themselves in this way. That his clothing choices – and their implications – have reached beyond his own neighbourhood presents Abdul with even more difficult terrain to navigate. He was never particularly safe venturing away from his home territory, but now he has as much to fear within his own neighbourhood as he does outside it.

During the team meeting, it was felt by all that Abdul might benefit from some mental-health intervention, as he has begun to show signs of anger and a tendency towards violence in his efforts to cope with the avalanche of social-media interest that the posted pictures have generated among young people – many of whom he knows, and many more he doesn't. Abdul has been referred to my clinic for support, but, before I can meet him, I need to see the photos that everyone is talking about.

'I don't think he's gay, though . . .' one of the youth workers says, as we continue to stand in front of the lifeless screen. 'You can't be gay and be in a gang,' he adds, for clarity, shaking his head.

Gangs are typically about money, territory, violence and identity, and this is how gang members invariably display their masculinity. They will usually be surrounded by materialistic girls and women who are drawn to them because of their power and bravado. To some girls, these gang members make great boyfriends because they will openly show affection, being unafraid to kiss in the middle of the street. To young women who know no better, this is their definition of what it is to be a man. But these displays are only to mark their territory. Once marked, the girls are obligated to run errands for them. In this version of society, there is no room for diverse sexuality.

'Well, if being gay means you're stigmatized, I would think a gang might be a good place to hide . . .' I suggest.

I catch Monty rolling his eyes. Clearly, despite my experience, I still don't fully understand how gangs work, and what I've suggested makes no sense to him. His time in prison will have informed his knowledge; prison itself, he has told me, is just an extension of the streets. The same rules apply. And being gay in prison is as challenging as being gay on the streets. There is no tolerance in either environment.

The first image appears. Abdul's tight pink shorts are figure-hugging. Riding high and snug. His hips jut forward, like a model posing for the cameras. His white shirt is cut high at the front, his belly button just visible above the waistband of the shorts. His hair is blown up into an afro, and perhaps there's a hint of glitter there, I can't quite tell. I peer harder at the screen.

He looks like someone from a hippie festival in the 1960s. But what strikes me most is that he looks happy. Proud of who he is. My instant reaction is to celebrate his clear sense of self, of freedom and liberty, but I can also see why this image has caused a fuss on the streets. I can better understand now why Abdul is worried.

In this first photo, Abdul is surrounded by what appear to be his friends. Some are girls. Others are older boys who might be in their early twenties. A few are younger, dressed in school uniforms. The team of youth workers seem to know all their names, as these are some of the young people in the borough who are at risk of being lured into gangs or are already in a gang. As I listen to them identify the crowd, I'm impressed. My highly skilled colleagues are an intelligence hub of their own and I love working with them and tapping into their extensive knowledge. But, while they debate the names of the young people in the picture, pointing to this one and that one, my eyes remain focused on Abdul.

Calvin presses a key and reveals a second picture. In this one, Abdul is wearing loose black trousers, like yoga pants. His belly is exposed again because he's topless, his hair held back by a bright bandana. He is positioned fully side-on this time, as though he's walking off, out of shot. The smile is gone. From the expression on his face, he seems distressed. The crowd around him has largely dispersed, leaving him more or less alone.

'I wonder if someone is forcing him to wear that stuff . . .' one of the youth workers suggests.

It's possible. Abdul, with his ADHD, is easy to pick on. He dropped out of school a long time ago. His dad works in a busy restaurant in the West End and his mother stays at home, sometimes selling Persian pottery at the market. Abdul comes from a solid, structured family, but ADHD and the lure of the streets have pulled him off track. The parental and community values that his mum and dad would be able to enforce if they were in Iran are much more difficult to put in place here in London. Western values promote individualism and freedom of expression. And while, as a society, we see this is a good thing, it can often conflict with the values of other cultures.

For Abdul's family, the behaviour of a son will be a matter of honour. And, as the oldest child, he's dutybound to carry forward the family name. All this is a lot for a young mind with ADHD to manage. And, in case that's not enough, Abdul is also asthmatic and refuses to carry his inhaler; at times, he can struggle for breath. The asthma, perceived as another weak link, is something that's bound to amuse the other kids.

'One for you, definitely, Nurse Dorcas,' I hear Mayse whisper, as we all edge forward to look even more closely at the new photo, trying to make sense of what it's telling us.

The youth workers know more than anyone about Abdul, and they share it all with me now, as part of the referral. I learn that he has been on the periphery of gangs for some time. He has been found in possession of cannabis several times. He has been seen among the following of a few of the more seasoned gang members, but he is by no means a leader. He was once caught stealing an expensive pair of women's high-heeled shoes from Selfridge's, which the youth workers think is an odd thing to do. It's possible that he might have stolen them to sell on. It's possible they were for his own use. His overall behaviour, they tell me, is not particularly out of character for a young person who is highly exposed to gangs. What is peculiar, given the context, is how overt he appears to be about his sexuality. And I can tell that the youth workers are just as perplexed as I am. I have never had a referral for a young person who is gay and exposed to gangs. The two worlds do not usually intersect. None of us has any real idea about what will happen next.

'My worry, Dorcas, is that the community is mocking Abdul.

They're ashamed of his behaviour – not his criminal behaviour, but his sexual behaviour,' Calvin says to me as we peel away from the laptop.

Abdul has taken to spending a lot of time with a boy called Ramel, a known hardcore gang member, and he seems to be doing this in order to distance himself from the rumours about his sexuality. He wants to prove to everyone that he isn't gay and that he can be as tough and as violent as the other boys, if not more so. Calvin tells me that, since the photos have surfaced and found their way to the wider community, Abdul's mum has been finding it hard to communicate with her son. The once strong mother–son bond is hanging by a thread and she doesn't know how to manage the emotions that have come with the weight of this information. When Calvin called her to talk about it, she repeatedly said, 'It's forbidden, it's forbidden, Calvin.' Homosexuality, she is adamant, is forbidden in their religion.

The intelligence shared by the youth workers is mesmerizing. Of all the professionals I work with, it's the youth workers who have had the greatest impact on me. Often having used the experience of prison to turn their own lives around, they are now committed to helping young people exposed to many of the same risk factors they once faced. It has been a steep learning curve for me, but my frontline nursing experience in the accident and emergency department lends itself well to working with the Gangs Unit. It's a chase that excites me – and it *is* a chase, because these young gang members never share the same compulsion to spend time with me. But to think that I can help them in some way keeps propelling me forward.

*

It's another week or so before Calvin and I are able to talk through Abdul's case again, this time in the canteen, where we catch up over a cup of coffee. I need to be clear about my objectives. What is it exactly that Calvin wants me to support Abdul with? And what kind of outcomes are we trying to achieve?

'Things are moving fast,' he tells me. 'It turns out Abdul is in a relationship with a girl from the estate. You might know her? She's definitely known to Mayse because she's quite vulnerable.'

Mayse has shared that the girl isn't known for any criminality, but that she comes from a fragile home, where it's just her and her mum. She has a speech disorder and has previously been known to child and adolescent mental-health services. It's all extremely useful knowledge to take with me. But the problem is this: Abdul has been verbally abusive to the girl, right from the start of the relationship, sometimes mocking her speech impairment. The verbal abuse is escalating and it appears the young girl has started to self-harm, making superficial cuts to her wrists. The girl has mentioned this abuse to Mayse, but she also wants to protect Abdul, so is ambivalent about going to A & E. This is common. The number of young women and girls who experience emotional abuse or physical violence from gang members and go on to press charges is low. I am not surprised by what I'm hearing.

'I think Abdul is doing this to show his masculinity and to prove to people that he couldn't possibly be gay, because he has a girl,' Calvin tells me.

He goes on to say what he needs from me to support the work he's already doing with Abdul.

'Talk to him about his anger, his frustration, the emotional abuse he's subjecting his girl to,' he tells me. 'And also check if this thing about him being gay is what's causing him to be so angry, because I know that can lead to violence, and if he needs help with that. Or whether it's something else.' He adds: 'We also need to check if his asthma is managed. His mum isn't really talking to him, but she still worries about him. And she isn't sure if he's carrying his inhalers with him.'

And, just like that, Abdul is a child again – a boy with health problems, who needs to be looked after.

Calvin thinks the best way for me to meet Abdul will be at his home, a late afternoon visit, as Abdul isn't really functioning until two or three. He thinks it might be good for me to meet his mum and gather more of the history from her, and perhaps try to support her too. She has many fears for her son, and not only about his sexuality and the challenges that presents. She's not happy that Abdul has been hanging out with Ramel. She is worried that Abdul will be stabbed, now that he's more involved with the gang. She's troubled that he is dating a white British girl from the estate, who comes from a single-parent home, rather than a girl from his own faith. And, given the latest development, that he could be arrested for domestic violence against this young girl who she wishes wasn't a part of his life.

Calvin has a good relationship with Abdul's mum and he wants me to build on that. He contacts her regularly and, although she doesn't speak much English, she's able to communicate her worries to him. And it's helpful that she has influence over Abdul's father. She is able to rein him in and facilitate a calm conversation about Abdul, however angry he is. Abdul's mum is the nucleus. She holds the family together. She is the key to my nursing interventions.

*

It's nearly four o'clock in the afternoon when I meet Calvin by a fish-and-chip shop on the edge of Abdul's estate. The sun is low in the sky. The busy main road is buzzing with schoolkids slowly making their way home, and many are lingering on the pavement outside the chip shop with me, hot food in their

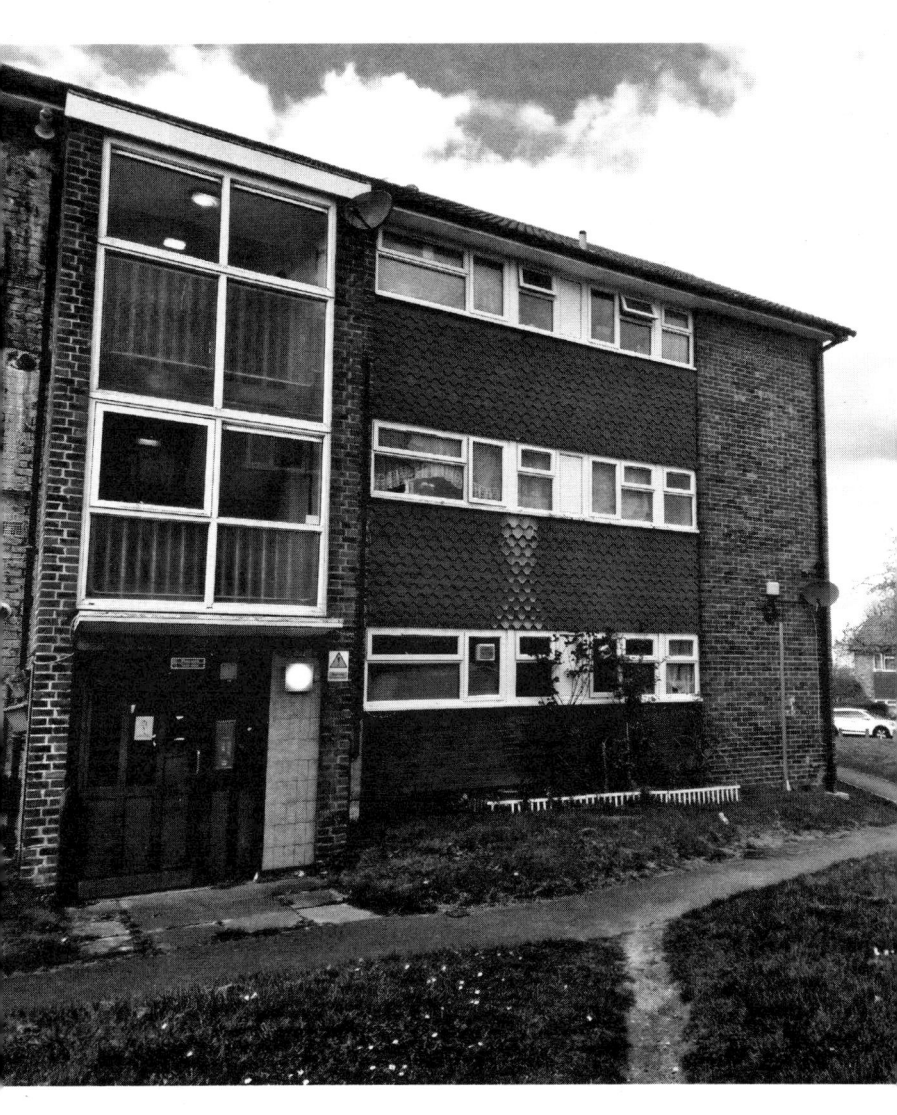

hands. A few girls dip in and out of the corner shop next door, their joyful screams lifting the dour atmosphere of the streets. I look closely to see if any of my clients are among them. They are not a menace to me. Unlike most people, I understand their vulnerability and I love to see them laughing with their friends and feeling good about life. I am more concerned about keeping my bike safe during the visit. I turn to the young people to help me.

'Auntie, no one's going to touch your bike,' they tell me. 'Leave it here. Anyone wants to touch your bike, they have to go through me.'

Somehow, true to their word, they keep it safe.

As I lock it up, Calvin hears from the mother that Abdul is not yet home. He's running late – or, quite possibly, avoiding us and the awkward conversation to come. We decide to press on without him. A few moments alone with his mother might prove useful.

The paintwork on Abdul's nineteen-storey building, dating from the late eighties, has faded in colour over the years. I know that the residents send frequent complaints to the council about the state of the ill-fitting windows which allow the wind to whistle through their homes, the dark walkways they fear to walk along and the unloved grassy areas that were supposed to provide community and make the urban setting less stark. The youth club used to offer some safety by shedding bright light onto the narrow pedestrian pathway that leads deep into the estate, but it was recently burned down in an incident of suspected arson, covered by the local news. Its dark carcass is all that remains, though teenagers still loiter outside its gates, as if attending a vigil for its loss. Three stabbings have taken place within its vicinity in the year since it closed. In one, a row had broken out between a boy known to our youth workers and another gang member from the same area but a different school. The quarrel quickly turned into a fist fight that spread to their friends and escalated into multiple stabbings and a fatality. I walk past the gates to the burned-out youth club with a heavy heart.

What do these young lads who hang out on the street corners make of Abdul's fashion fiasco? They have probably mocked him mercilessly. They will have given him a brutal nickname, a gay slur, which will be hard to shake off. What most likely started as a bit of a joke has escalated into painful humiliation and a spiral of anxiety for the victim, which may lead to social isolation, self-harm or retaliatory violence. With social media amplifying the problem, Abdul's world has changed and it's hard to imagine that it will ever be the same again. While he has been able to control some elements on the streets by making certain associations, he has no control over the digital platforms which are the focus of so many eyes. I wonder how his mental health is holding up, given the frightening pressures. I hope that we are about to find out.

At the building's surprisingly solid front door, we press the bell for Abdul's flat. A soft voice answers. Abdul's mother, Leila, buzzes us into a bleak foyer with a dauntingly dim stairwell in one corner. We take the solitary lift, the smell of urine filling our nostrils as we press the button for the twelfth floor. As we wait for the lift to shudder into action, Calvin and I have a moment to collect ourselves. It's usual on these family visits for the youth worker to focus on the young person while I gain the mum's trust. We both know the drill.

We knock on Abdul's front door and a middle-aged woman dressed in a black abaya opens it and welcome us in. Her manner is as conservative as her dress and I'm careful to offer her every respect. We take our shoes off in the hallway, as per custom, and step into the living room. The home is immaculately clean, with warm-toned Iranian rugs scattered across the living-room floor,

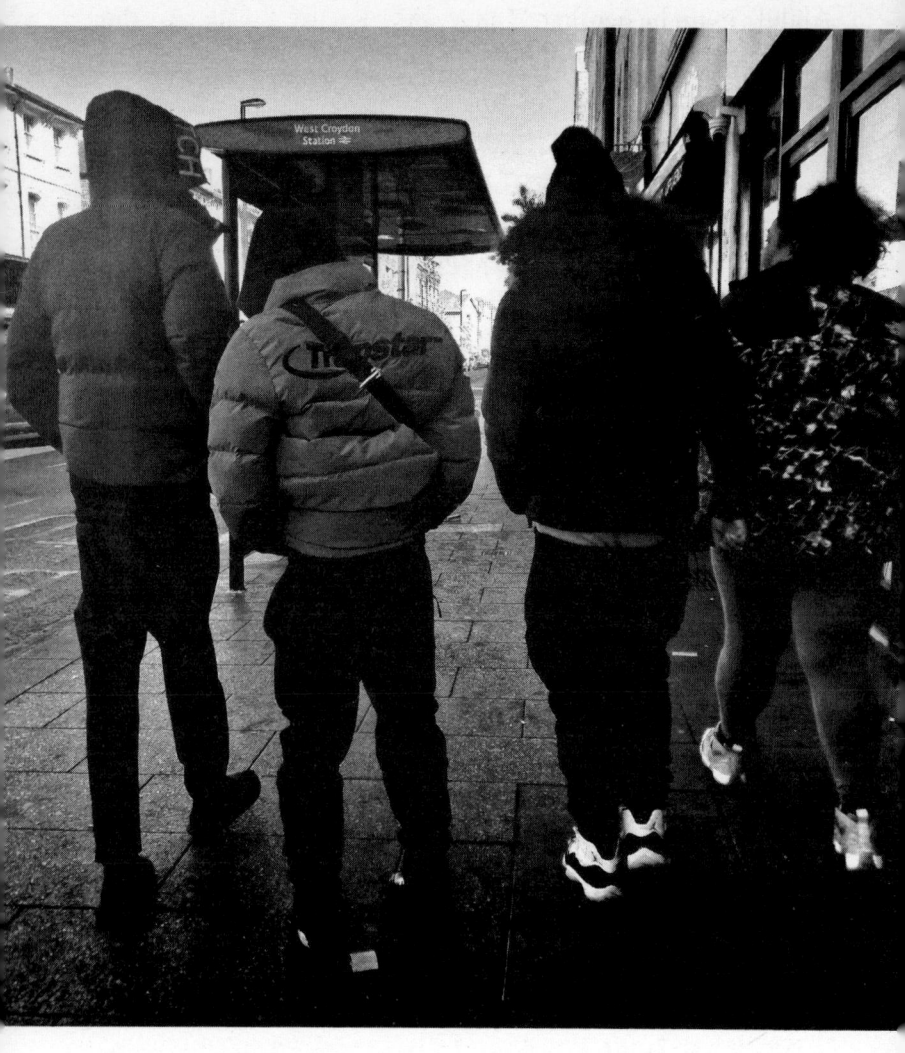

where we're encouraged to sit. Clearly comfortable, Calvin calls Abdul's mum by her first name.

'Leila, I've come with my colleague Nurse Dorcas today,' he says, gesturing towards me by way of introduction.

'Salam,' I greet her.

Leila speaks Farsi, not Arabic. The two languages, though they have some similarities, are distinctly different. While I have a little conversational Arabic, my Farsi is non-existent. But Leila, I know, won't be concerned about the accuracy or otherwise of my cultural greetings. Right now, she is overwhelmed by other thoughts.

Our eyes meet. I'm a nurse, not a social worker, and that is going to work in my favour. For families such as Leila's, social workers represent the law – the law that takes children away from their parents. Doctors are trusted slightly more than social workers, but their care is hard to come by; very few doctors will visit families like Leila's at home or see them in the streets. Leila needs to know that I am here to work with her, not against her.

As we round up our greetings, I hear the front door click open then slam shut. Footsteps come our way. Abdul emerges from the narrow hallway, a little out of breath, as if he has been running. He's an imposing young man, slimmer in the flesh than in the photographs. The sides of his head are shaved, giving rise to a flop of hair on his forehead. I can tell he's a little stressed about having all four of us in this small space, and it bothers him that we have arrived before him. He feels the need to take control of the conversation. For any young person, there are some things they just don't want their mum to know, and that's particularly the case for Abdul. It's partly to protect her, but it's also about trying to gain some autonomy. Calvin knows this too, so he jumps in.

'Alright, bruv.' He greets Abdul with a smile.

They shake hands, engaging in a half-hug, like sportsmen on the field. Their conversation, I note, is half street and half formal English, sliding effortlessly between the two. The interaction is organic and authentic, embedded in trust and respect. Calvin offers Abdul positive feedback about turning up for the Safer Neighbourhood event that was recently run by the council. Abdul teases Calvin about his bald head, brushing his fingers lightly across Calvin's sleek skull. Calvin ducks out of the way and, for a moment, they are just two playful young men, the city that has no respect for either of them receding.

'Hi, I am Nurse Dorcas.' I introduce myself to Abdul as he peels himself away from the tussle.

'You alright, Nurse,' he says to me, not looking for an answer.

So that they can talk, Abdul takes Calvin into his bedroom, the only place he probably feels he has any privacy. He is lucky. Many of the young people I work with don't have a bedroom of their own. Most have to share with siblings, or other relatives, meaning bunk beds are common, with the older siblings setting the tone and establishing the rules and regulations of how to be in that space. But, regardless of overcrowding, the bedroom – or even just their own bed – remains a sacred space for young people, somewhere they can be in control, in a world in which they often feel powerless.

Leila and I are left in the living room. With Calvin gone, she becomes more curious about me and begins to probe. I am used to these questions, never fighting them. This is where engagement with a patient begins to happen, or not. And, once the rules of engagement are established, Leila and I can move on to the issues at hand.

She says, 'I am worried, Doco.'

As ever, I don't attempt to correct my name; it's enough that she is prepared to open up to me, a stranger in her home. As she speaks, she leads us into the kitchen, which is also immaculately clean and tidy. Here, without drapes across the windows, the view from the twelfth floor is breathtaking. I make out the edges of the burned-out Grenfell Tower to the west and, to the east, the BT Tower in central London. It's late afternoon and the lights in the buildings are just coming on, illuminating a spectacular view of the whole city. I breathe in the calmness and quiet that in London you can only get at this height. Forcing myself to look away from the window, I turn back to Leila, who is making us a cup of Persian tea. The ritualistic process is equally soothing.

'Doco, did you see the pictures? They say Abdul is gay. He is dressed like a woman. This is haram in our religion.' Leila shakes her head. 'It's haram,' she says again, in an agitated voice. She waves her hands around, the teaspoon punctuating the air with exclamation marks. For Leila, homosexuality isn't two individuals enjoying each other or falling in love. It's more likely to be viewed solely through the act of sex. In certain cultures, where the belief is that sex can only take place between members of different sexes, the idea of homosexuality is difficult to comprehend. This is the case in many countries in the world. And when we're unable to understand something, we too often seek to ban it.

'Doco, now, because of those pictures, everybody is talking,' she adds in a subdued voice.

As her distress deepens, there's a wheeziness to her breathing. Like many parents with an adolescent they're unable to keep safe, Leila's own health problems are worsened by the stress she's living with. Managing Abdul's behaviour is putting a massive strain on her body. Hypertension and asthma are troubling her.

'Leila, what do *you* think about the pictures?' I ask her gently.

'I think nothing. It's forbidden in our religion. I don't want anyone talking about it because it is haram.' She stops for a moment and draws breath as she pours hot water into a shining gold-coloured teapot. 'Anyway, Abdul has a girlfriend now. I don't like the girl myself, but it shows you that he is not gay.'

That Leila is against homosexuality is clear, but I still don't know if, despite her strong reservations about diverse sexuality, she is willing to believe that her son might be gay and, if so, accept him for what he is. I am treading carefully and one wrong word could break this intimate new relationship before it's fully formed. But I have to keep going with my line of enquiry.

'What do you not like about the girl?' I ask Leila.

'She is not a Muslim. I know the family. Everyone knows that family. They are British,' she tells me. 'She is a nice girl, don't get me wrong. Very nice. But I am not sure if she is the one for Abdul.'

Leila pours the aromatic tea into tiny bulb-shaped cups. I add half a teaspoon of brown sugar to mine and stir. As she does the same, Leila is lost momentarily in thought.

'Doco, every mother wants the best for their child,' she says eventually. 'Abdul was a difficult child for me. From birth, it was difficult. His father was in Iran when he was born; I was alone. Then he came back. Abdul and me, we're very close. He has always looked out for Mummy. I have to look out for him, too. But it is hard.'

I realize now that her sense of her son is a world away from that of our youth workers who know Abdul from the streets, and who know that, as he becomes increasingly caught up on the periphery of gang culture, he is as dangerous as he is vulnerable. How is it possible to square these two opposing sides of the same person?

We hear the bedroom door open; Abdul is in conversation with Calvin, their voices growing louder as they move towards the living room, where Leila and I have now settled with our tea. In their company, she doesn't make an attempt to repeat the agitated words she directed to me. I realize she feels safer voicing her objections to me about Abdul's possible sexuality, and to his choice of girlfriend, than she does to her own son.

'Abdul, I really want you to catch up with Nurse Dorcas this week,' Calvin says. 'She wants to have a chat with you about your asthma and about how you're feeling. Would that be OK, bruv?' His tone is caring but insistent. He doesn't want to leave any choice in the matter. With compassion, he is persuading Abdul to take the help on offer, making it clear that he thinks it's in Abdul's best interests.

'Yeah, sure, man, sure,' Abdul says with studied casualness.

*

I arrange to catch up with Abdul at the local education centre, which doubles as a makeshift youth club three nights a week, managing to secure a room to meet with him privately. I don't want what will be an intimate conversation about his moods, feelings and sexuality to be overheard by anyone else. The stakes are too high; Abdul could be further persecuted and would lose trust in me.

He arrives at twenty past three in the afternoon, twenty minutes past our appointment time, and my response is to be accommodating, patient, forgiving. He is wearing a pair of skinny black jeans, a white T-shirt and a hooded sweatshirt that covers half his face. I notice that he is much more anxious today. He greets me politely and I see that his eyes are slightly unfocused – most likely the after-effects of cannabis use. I let it go. He is here.

As we settle down, there's a knock on the door. Through the glass, I can see it's another young person. I ease the door open a crack and the boy peers in, finding Abdul with his eyes.

'Ramel, I'm coming, man. Let me speak to the nurse,' Abdul whispers.

The door closes again.

'That's my friend Ramel, innit,' Abdul explains to me, although no explanation is needed.

Abdul's attention is now torn between me and his friend. Like so many of my patients, he is in a constant rush, his attention pushed and pulled in different directions at all times, and it's even more of a problem for someone with ADHD. I can see that Abdul is hyperactive and impulsive, ready to spring out of his chair at any moment, and yet he is also sensitive, with a hunger to please the professionals around him, as well as friends like Ramel. It's a character trait which makes him easy prey for gang members.

In the wake of the rumours about Abdul's sexuality, Ramel has challenged the gossipers. Not so much to defend Abdul, but to protect himself; he cannot be dragged into a debate about homosexuality. And, in Ramel's somewhat simplistic view, there is no way Abdul, a friend of his, could be gay. Ramel intends to prove this by pulling Abdul deeper into gang life, where his masculinity can be showcased through violence, performed to help redefine gang territory and enforce the gang's strict hierarchy. Once proven, according to Ramel's way of thinking, all gossip about his friend will go away. Calvin has told me that Ramel is trying to move Abdul up the ranks. Leila is right. It's a turn of events that has the potential to cost Abdul his life.

Abdul suddenly seems weary. He slumps down lower in the chair, but manages a half-smile in my direction.

I return it. 'How are you?' I enquire.

'Yeah, I'm alright. But I am stressed, though,' Abdul says.

His willingness to be open with me catches me off-guard.

'What are you most stressed about?' I ask him.

I assume Calvin has told Abdul that I've seen the pictures that went viral, and that I know about the issues with his new girlfriend. But I am keen to hear Abdul articulate these problems himself. He is at the heart of the challenges, and also at the heart of the solutions.

Of all his problems, which, I want to know, is his priority?

'The stuff about the pictures is still bothering me,' Abdul eventually says, eyes now averted.

I nod. 'What else is bothering you?' I ask gently, my voice only just above a whisper.

I want to bring calm to the room. I want Abdul to feel safe and at ease. I am working to carve out a therapeutic environment by seeking eye contact and providing reassurance. I want Abdul to feel understood so that he's able to express his thoughts and feelings freely, knowing that he can do so without judgement. Abdul has faced discrimination and rejection from many people around him, including people he loves. He needs to know that he will not face it here.

He takes a while to think about his response.

'I've got problems with this girl that I'm seeing,' he says. 'Well, my family has a problem with her, not me. And I got stopped by the police for just a piece of joint, and they're trying to make it like a big thing, innit. That's stressing me out as well.'

'Anything else?' I encourage him.

'Nah, that's it. That's why my friend is helping me, innit. He's helping me, innit,' he repeats. It's a verbal tic employed to reinforce understanding, one that I've observed in a lot of my young people who have learning difficulties, and all the more so when they are trying to make sense of their fears.

I pause and allow for some silence in the room, a moment for reflection. But the silence is shattered by Ramel, who is back, knocking at the door. This time, it's Abdul who gets up to speak to his friend and to set some boundaries. This is his time and, to my delight, he wants to claim it.

'I'm just with the nurse. I'll call when I'm finished, yeah?' he says to Ramel, with barely suppressed impatience. He quietly closes the door on his friend.

Through the glass, I see Ramel walk towards the exit, followed by a group of young people, many of them school age. A modern-day Pied Piper.

Abdul seems relieved to see the back of him. But, given some time to focus on himself, he also appears to be overwhelmed by it all. He is fidgety and unsettled in the chair. I reach for my problem-solving skills, which are rooted in cognitive behavioural therapy. I need to understand the effect that Abdul's social environment is having on his physical and mental wellness, and to be clear about which of his needs he perceives to be a priority.

'Out of those three challenges, which one do you think is the biggest for you?' I ask him.

Abdul inhales slowly. 'It's the same thing, innit? It's all mashed up together,' he says through a long sigh. Then, he speaks in a rush, suddenly animated: 'I don't know why a man has to defend himself because he's wearing pink. So what if I was wearing them pink pants? Don't mean nothing!' he protests.

This, clearly, is the biggest problem that Abdul is facing.

'Miss, if you go to the Middle East, or even in Africa, yeah, men hug each other all the time. They kiss each other all the time. That don't mean nothing,' he continues.

He is correct, of course. Culturally, it means nothing more than friendship and respect, or platonic love. But I need to know what it means for him.

'Abdul, are you gay?' I ask him outright.

His eyes, which have been flitting around the room, turn to focus on me. He is shaking a little, I notice, and, as he searches for his words, I can tell his mouth is dry.

'Miss, around here, man's not allowed to be gay,' he says evenly.

Abdul isn't answering my question, and I can only imagine how difficult it would be for him to say those words, or even to think them. Instead, he's communicating something between the lines: fear and anger. Both of which spring from living in a social context that is as complex as his own sexuality. But, even within this complexity, Abdul has rights. I want to fight for his right to express himself freely, to live his own life, on his own terms.

'What do you think about gay people, Miss?' Abdul asks me.

He is testing the waters. I am cautious about sharing my views; this is about Abdul, not about me. But it's a good question. He wants to know if it's safe enough in this room for him to reveal his true self. And he's right to challenge me. After all, I'm part of the very community that is now challenging him. The NHS provides us with many policies and guidelines on equality and inclusion, however patient experiences of the system are varied, and the system is not free of prejudice. Beyond the four walls of our safe space, Abdul and I know that gay people are being persecuted and their human rights violated. You don't have to travel as far as Uganda or Jamaica, where I've seen horrific persecution, to bear witness to that hatred.

London, though, has the ability to absorb diversity. It's a place of both individualism and community, and it's possible to flourish here despite and sometimes because of that diversity. But this is not necessarily true for my clients. To live on a council estate in London can sometimes be more like living in downtown Kingston, Nairobi or even Tehran. There are places where the right of freedom of expression is not afforded. Rather, how you're allowed to express yourself is determined by the culture of the streets where you live. There, homosexuality, I have learned, is rarely accepted, and certainly not from people of colour. Over the years, I have met a number of gay people of colour who have been ostracized by their families, many finding new friends and forming new families elsewhere, away from their community. Others, who aren't able to move away, are forced to live in isolation.

I am reminded of the gay African man from Nigeria who I looked after in A & E. He was anxious and depressed because his mother was at the end of her life and his sexuality meant he couldn't go to the funeral in Nigeria for fear of being killed. And of the young woman from Pakistan who sought refuge in the UK after disclosing her sexuality to her family. Her uncle's response had been to order her killing. Although she had found comfort and safety among the queer community in London, she still lived in fear. I can't help but think about a Brazilian client who was ostracized by his Catholic family because of his sexuality.

I have long tested people's tolerance within my own community, where homosexuality is often discussed in terms of fear and hostility. I won't shy away from posing the question to parents about what they would do if their child disclosed that they were gay. The question alone is enough to arouse tempers. 'Not in my house!' many will say.

I press pause on our conversation and introduce Abdul to my 'Mood and Feelings' questionnaire, which I hold in my head. First, I ask him about his sleep, a significant indicator for low mood. He tells me that he typically sleeps from around 4 a.m. to just after midday, but that his sleep is disrupted by anxious thoughts and bad dreams. We explore feelings of anger, frustration, violence and guilt. I am particularly curious to talk about this latter emotion with Abdul, as I'm wondering if he's self-blaming about the impact the pictures have had on his family. Does he feel bad about shattering the family's image within the community, knowing how much the community loves to gossip? And I explore the psychological effects that the images have had on his own mental health. He is open with his feelings; he tells me that he's trying to remove the images from his mind. However, despite his efforts, he often finds himself thinking about it all again. He mentions that, when he does, he feels panicked, sweaty, and has trouble breathing. He experiences some nausea and a pounding heart. Abdul, speaking freely now, tells me about the social anxiety that he has been experiencing. It's as if, he says, the streets are watching him. It makes him wary, on guard.

Taking a non-judgemental approach, I allow Abdul to express his truth as he works through what he thinks and feels. As his nurse, I want to assure him that I embrace his and others' diversity in the most human way.

The questions are rated one to five, with five being the highest score. Abdul scores at the top end of the range on many questions, such as how he's sleeping, and he also scores highly on poor concentration and low mood – so much so, I ask if he has recently had any thoughts of suicide or thoughts of harming others. In our mental-health assessments we rely on what the patient tells us as much as what we observe, always aware that some patients may not say much and that this may be a function of their depression. Our objective view of the patient's behaviour provides a more comprehensive analysis; it makes sense to use our own observations to assess risk. Abdul pauses before answering, then says he has not been feeling suicidal. But I don't rely solely on what Abdul tells me. Clinically, his speech is flat, and his mind seems to be overrun with flashbacks of the pictures and the wildfire they caused. My clinical observation is factual but it is also compassionate.

Mentally, I switch to my 'Impact of Events' questionnaire. I want to know how the photographs and the sharing of them has affected him. Abdul tells me that it has been a dark time for him, as traumatic as the time he was chased by a group of boys who intended to stab him. Although he can briefly put it all out of his mind, reality all too quickly kicks back in, and he is reminded again of the mockery and gay slurs. He feels as though the whole estate is scrutinizing his clothing, looking out for any feminine behaviours which they can leap on and use against him.

My role as his nurse is to advocate for him and provide the environment to allow him to express his feelings. This evidenced-based examination gives me a feel for Abdul's current mental state. He assures me that he doesn't have any thoughts of harming himself, but he wishes it would all go away. On balance, I get the sense that Abdul simply wants acceptance from those around him, acceptance of himself and his choices; and he wants validation and emotional support from his parents – his mother, in particular. I take some time to think through how to structure my next conversation with his mother, who's so key to his safety and mental-health development. And then I change tack.

'Are you seeing someone at the moment?' I ask him.

There is no pleasure in his eyes as he thinks about his girlfriend. 'Yeah, but it's complicated,' he replies dully.

'What's complicated?' I ask him, although of course I know something of the issues already. 'Are you using any protection when you have sex?'

It's an important question that I ask all my young people. Often, they giggle and brush it away. Some deny that they're having sex at all. Others brag about the sex they're not actually having. While many parents in my communities panic at the idea of their children having sex in their early adolescence – and most forbid it, or at least try to – my conversations with young people always start with, 'Are you having safe sex?' rather than, 'Why are you having sex?' It is the biggest taboo in many of my families: the thing we don't talk about, and where thick lines of morality are drawn. Society the world over is brutally judgemental, and a sexually active man is not viewed through the same lens as a sexually active woman.

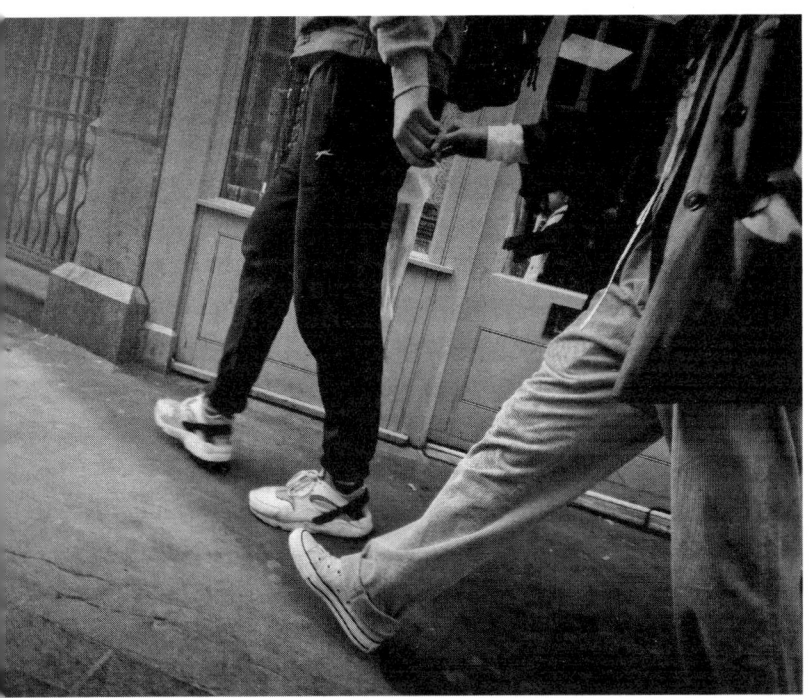

'I'm using condoms, innit.' Abdul laughs out loud, his head thrown back, his teeth on show. He is tickled by our conversation. It is, if nothing else, good to see him smile.

'Is it serious, then? Do you love her?' I probe him.

'It's not like that. You don't understand,' he replies quickly. 'That's the thing. Everywhere I turn, people are saying, "You can't do this, you can't do that." My family are saying that we can't be together because she's not the girl they would have chosen for me.'

Abdul is confused, caught between two worlds. He doesn't know what to think. No wonder he is struggling to breathe.

'What does Calvin think?' I ask.

'Man, if it wasn't for Calvin, I wouldn't have survived this, you know. He has really helped me. Especially when I was feeling so violent and angry I wanted to punch someone. I wanted to stab someone, innit,' Abdul admits.

I nod. Again, I am in awe of what our youth workers do, their ability to engage with some of the most excluded young people in our society, those on the fringes of serious criminal activity, who will take their lives in the wrong direction if left to their own devices. Calvin and his colleagues have an insatiable appetite for keeping young people safe and out of crime. Whatever Calvin believes about homosexuality, he cares deeply about Abdul and all his young clients.

What I'm seeing here are signs of clinical anxiety. There is no doubt in my mind that Abdul is stressed. His use of cannabis to cope with that stress is counterproductive; all it does is exacerbate his anxiety. After just twenty-five minutes talking with him, it's quite clear that there needs to be an intervention.

Before I can respond, a thump on the door tells us that Ramel is back again, unable to keep to the arrangement that Abdul tried to put in place. He is impatient in his manner now, as though an emergency has arisen and Abdul is needed. Our conversation is over.

'I have to go, innit,' Abdul says to me as he stands up.

I want to bring a tidy closure to the session, but Ramel is in a rush.

'Thanks for talking to me,' I say. 'Can we catch up next week, on Tuesday afternoon?'

'Text me, innit, otherwise I'll forget,' he shouts over his shoulder as he leaves the room.

From the doorway, I watch Abdul bump fists with several of the other young people. With Ramel around, he is confident now and stands tall. He shoves his hood over his head, Ramel pushes the doors open, and they both disappear into the streets, entourage in tow.

*

A few days later, I call Abdul's mother from the office for a catch-up.

'Doco, my dear,' Leila says. Her voice sounds shallow, but she rushes on with what she wants to tell me. 'I don't care what Abdul chooses, I just want him to be safe and to do well. My husband the same. We want him to be safe, that's all.'

It's clear that Abdul's parents have been doing some tough thinking – fearful of losing their relationship with their son, perhaps, or they've simply come to their senses.

I see an opportunity to enter into a therapeutic discussion about how Leila can reconcile with Abdul on a deep, emotional level. I know accepting that a child is gay can be difficult, especially if the parents hold differing values around sex and sexuality. Researcher Apoorva Ghosh has explored the experiences of young gay and lesbian people in traditional heteronormative families and has outlined that acceptance may take time; the process of transitioning to acceptance can be complex and may require access to counselling or therapy. Having supportive friends or extended family is also helpful.

In some ways, Abdul has already come out. He has been laid bare across the internet in photos that have lit touchpapers among his friends and across the neighbourhood. After the initial shock, it is now time for his parents and the community to accept him, and Leila has a key role to play. As the matriarch of the family, she can provide the emotional connection that the family needs, and, if she is accepting, then Abdul's father is, in time, more likely to come on board.

Leila shares with me her fears for Abdul. She had dreams for him, that he would grow up and do well, get a job and marry a nice girl from their background and faith.

'That's all I want for him,' she tells me. 'That's all.'

I can hear Leila breathing softly down the phone line, regulating her breaths as if in meditation, taking this moment in, being mindful of it. We talk through how she can reconnect with Abdul. If he feels safe in his home environment, then he may not feel the need to be violent and antisocial outside the home. Once he feels accepted and embraced by the people he loves, he'll better be able to form healthy relationships with people who will ensure his safety, rather than seeking refuge among gang members who are invariably violent and territorial. Leila needs to reclaim her son from the gangs. I encourage her to take steps to spend quality time with Abdul, to knock on his bedroom door and seek out conversations, be intentional about attending family events together, and to provide the kind of emotional presence which shows unconditional love. This journey of acceptance and psychological safety is underpinned by love.

Leila makes the point that her and her husband accepting Abdul is not enough; Abdul has to make the right choices in life, to keep himself safe and avoid behaviours that will get him arrested and criminalized. I acknowledge this and assure her that Calvin will be picking this up with Abdul. He too has work to do.

As I round off my conversation with Leila, I commend her for the courage and compassion she has resolutely displayed in the face of the family's difficulties. I am hopeful that she is not merely saying the words of acceptance but actively transforming her thoughts and feelings towards Abdul. Above all, I hope Abdul learns that, in order to live well as someone who is different, the solution is not to resort to violence and domination in an attempt to avoid the pertinent issues. I hope he learns to face his issues, however complex.

3. Lori: The Cafe

'Minoritised women from particular contexts and communities are more likely to be criminalised, viewed as complicit in violence towards them and thus less likely to be considered "victims" of sexual violence.'

LORI LIVES IN THE south-east of the borough, but the mainstream clinic, which she should attend, is based in the north-west. We know from experience that, for safety reasons, young people exposed to gang violence and exploitation can struggle to travel across postcodes. So, given my flexible community-engagement approach and my experience in family therapy and youth violence, the clinic staff feel it would be best if Lori is referred via the Gangs Unit to my street clinic, so that I can come to her whenever suits her, and wherever she feels safe. Her referral note says little more than that she is a sixteen-year-old child from a vulnerable background and she is a victim of sexual assault.

After receiving the referral, I quickly send Lori a number of text messages, communicating with her using the method she and most young people prefer. No letters. No email. It doesn't take long for us to agree on a time and place for our first session, and we meet in a cafe on a surprisingly quiet street a few minutes' walk from a teeming central-London Tube station.

Lori seems to feed off our combined energy, her elegant fingers with their polished nails tracing the strands of her braids as she extends them, over and over, to their full length, then allows them to bounce back into their natural shape. It's pleasing to see her claiming her place in a new generation of young women who embrace their natural hair, leaning into their cultural identity even in the face of pressures from social media to look a certain way. It's a pressure that can also come from young men, who want to determine and control the identity of their girlfriends, making them adhere to their own perception of beauty. Lori, I instantly note, has a strong sense of self.

Our first session is exploratory, with Lori weighing up the likely value to her of the sessions. Can she trust me? Can our therapeutic relationship build her up and allow her to walk away from her trauma? Or is she wasting her time? Am I wasting her time? The young people and their families with whom I work have a way of analysing the professionals assigned to help them that is both efficient and brutal. Many do not trust easily, and with good reason. They try to look through you and into your soul, searching your very core for evidence of either authenticity or deceit. I am very aware of this in my first interaction with Lori. She is doing her research.

Nurses generally have a good social contract with society. They are mostly trusted, and seen as a constant where other professionals are merely intermittent, coming and going. I don't take this trust for granted. Rather, I leverage it, fusing it with the skills I've gained from various areas of my work, including the global-health field, to gain young people's trust and engagement.

Very quickly, Lori and I are able to connect on a therapeutic level. I share with her just the right amount of information about my background in nursing and my wider experience, which often helps to strengthen the bond of trust. And, from the outset, I am clear about the nurse–patient relationship requiring boundaries. She takes it all in, and she understands.

That first meeting, I ask Lori about her own background and she tells me that her mother's side of the family are originally from Jamaica, and that her mother named her after her own mother, Lorraine, whom everybody calls Ms Lori. Ms Lori moved back to Jamaica a couple of years ago, but Lori doesn't feel particularly connected to the wider family there; much as she misses her grandmother and wants to visit her, she has no idea how to make that happen.

I ask Lori what she loves most about her grandmother, and she talks at length, with a new spark in her eyes, about how she likes her grandmother's cooking, her rice and peas and curry goat especially. She's keen to tell me that she loves how her nan relates everything to what she knows best; she would always say, 'Back home in Jamaica . . .' or, 'When I was a young girl growing up in Jamaica . . .' to help tell a story, to make a point, and to make sense of the very different world in which she now lived.

'What I love most about her, though,' Lori goes on, 'is that she always stood up for me. She would defend my corner. When me and Mum were at each other's throats, Nan would stand up for me. I love her for that.'

Lori doesn't know who her father is and her mother never discusses it; that is a conversation Lori feels her mother will never be ready to have. I can tell that Lori is gently probing to see how much she can share privately in our session, and how much of what she tells me might get back to her mum.

All professionals working with vulnerable groups are bound by confidentiality, and nurses are no exception. It is comprehensively covered in the Code of Ethics for Nurses. For those of us working with young people below the age of eighteen, the boundaries of confidentiality are not limited to the young person alone, and we always inform the young person that we

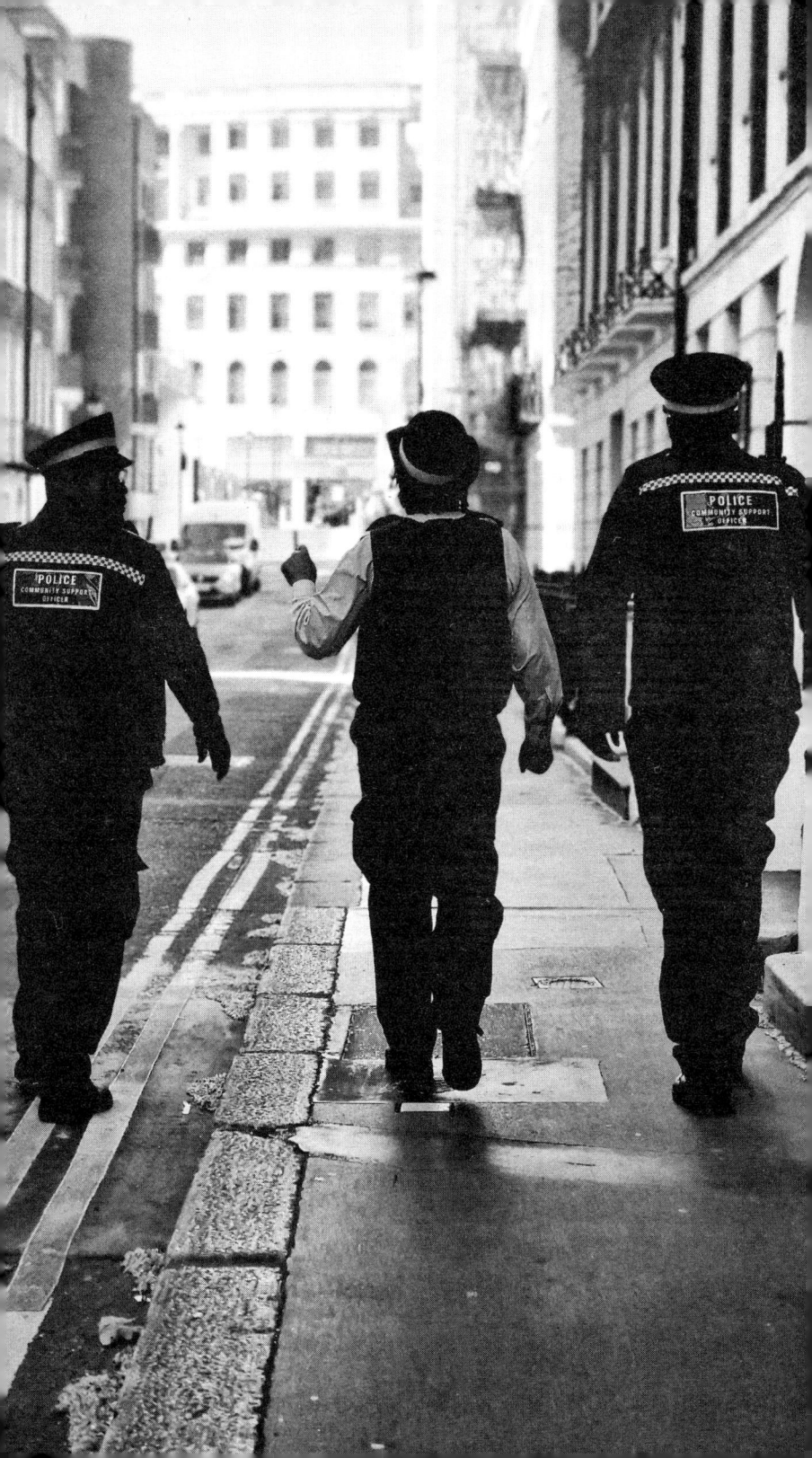

do need to share information with their parents or guardians. Many will already be familiar with the boundaries of confidentiality through their contact with other agencies, such as the police, social services and education. Young people are usually comfortable with this. Often, the young people I work with are more concerned about the information they share getting back to other young people than they are about it getting back to their parents.

Some young people who have had problems with trust – whether with their families or professionals – may want to be reassured of a degree of confidentiality at the beginning of their relationship with a nurse or therapist. Mostly, they want to know that I'm not a police officer disguised as a nurse, because, often, their relationship with the police is problematic. They also want to be sure that I am not a conduit for news or gossip between gangs, which would potentially put them at risk. Gangs maintain a high-level intelligence network, where information travels swiftly to those at the top. Words said in private can all too easily make their way to the wrong ears, and the young people I typically work with – who, along with everything else, are frequently facing neurodiversity challenges such as learning difficulties, autism, dyslexia and poor literacy skills – can be unaware of how far the network's tentacles reach.

Lori, I learn, doesn't have any neurodivergence. She admits to having smoked cannabis a handful of times, as many young people do, but seems to have no real interest in it and the habit has tailed off. Nonetheless, she is vulnerable, and she wears her vulnerability on her sleeve. Perhaps the ordinary Londoner passing her on the street wouldn't notice the self-harm marks on her legs or that her heavy make-up masks the bruises from occasional street fights with other girls struggling to survive on the periphery of gang life. She might not be one to walk past a fight or to avoid conflict, but she is unlikely to start a fight herself.

Lori tells me that her mother has taught her in no uncertain terms that, if another girl disrespects her or comes into her space or tries to take something that is hers, she should stand up for herself with her words and with her fists, because this is what her mother did in her time.

Over the years, Lori has been involved in a number of street fights with other girls, mostly over boys that the girls fancied and wanted to claim as their own, and sometimes over careless gossip, words said that couldn't then be unsaid. In the last fight she had, the rival girls from the estate across the road from her own had cornered her as she walked back from school alone. They jumped on her, pulling her hair until clumps came away in their fists and ripping her clothes at the seams. They punched her on every part of her body, drawing bruises that marked her for weeks. Lori put up a fight, just like her mother had taught her, grabbing one of the girls by the hair and dragging her across the pavement. As she did so, the biggest girl in the group kicked Lori hard in the face, her heavy boot leaving a deep cut on Lori's soft skin, blood pouring from her nose. With adrenalin pumping, Lori fought on wildly. Then, despite the rushing noise in her head and the *whoomph-whoomph* of her fast-beating heart, she heard the voice of an adult shouting: 'Stop! Stop it! You'll kill that poor girl!' The sound of a police siren made the gang of girls scatter every which way across the housing estate.

Lori had hoped her mother would arrive at the scene before the police, quietly taking her home to tend to her wounds. Instead, as her face began to swell, the police – one male, one female – arrived on the scene. They showed compassion, aware of their duty to safeguard young people, as well as their duty to enforce the law. But they probed her for the identities of the girls who had attacked her. Lori knew better than to name names. That was the street code you abided by, no matter what.

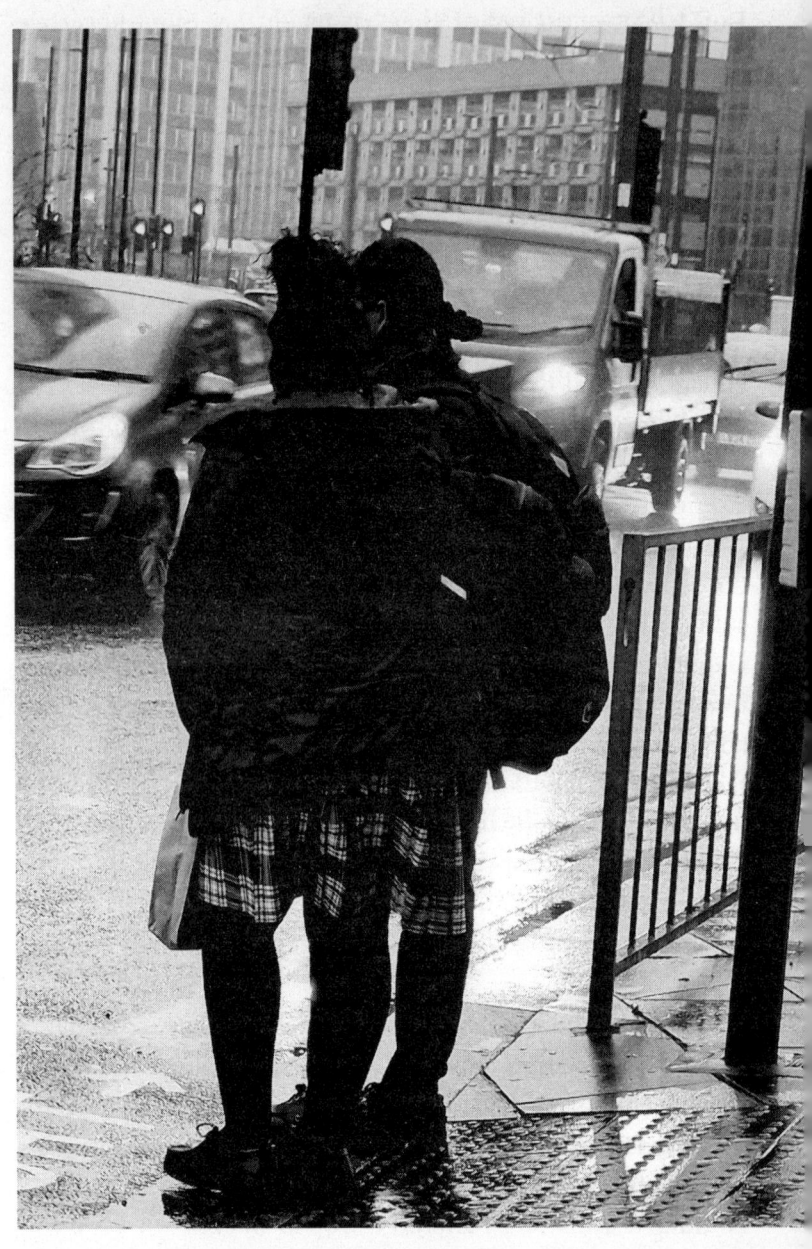

But somehow the police knew the names of the girls anyway and dropped them into conversation, while Lori tried not to react. The ambulance arrived, saving her from further interrogation and delivering her into what she perceived as more caring hands. When her mother appeared, Lori thought that she would be proud of her for standing up for herself. Instead, she ridiculed her for walking back from school alone despite knowing the dangers that existed around the estate, for not being quick enough to get away from the girls, for not being strong enough to fend them off, for allowing them to disrespect her. She didn't ask Lori how she felt. She didn't attempt to comfort her. Since then, Lori has learned to take her problems elsewhere. Talking to her mum is not an option.

Thinking that her mother might help her had been a foolish hope. Though she got it wrong that time, Lori is pretty self-sufficient. She learned to rely on herself from a young age. She's learned to judge risk, especially from other girls. She's learned to vary the times she walks back from school and is careful about the postcodes she crosses. She does her research before talking to any boy, knowing now that a friendly chat can lead to a fight with a girl who sees her as a rival. Lori has learned to guard herself against the many risks that other girls pose. But she's been unable to protect herself against the boys.

*

It's nine o'clock in the morning and, deep in the bowels of the Underground station, crowds of people are teeming around me. I step off a busy Tube and onto a chaotic platform in search of the Victoria Line. Everywhere I look, passengers are criss-crossing each other's paths, each focused on their own personal journey. Nothing else matters. I am just a drop in an ocean that is filling up fast with people furiously intent on getting to wherever they need to be. As I take off in what I hope is the right direction,

London's heartbeat pounds in my ears – the sound of rhythmic footfall accompanied by the swaying of bodies, the *swoosh* of the Tube doors opening and closing. Time is not on my side. I'm running late for my 9.30 a.m. therapy session with Lori, and the etiquette is that a good therapist turns up long before the client.

Unlike the young men I work with in my street clinic, Lori has chosen morning sessions with me; she has no trouble getting up and her days are fairly structured. And, unlike the boys, Lori is always on time. I am usually on time too; the unspoken rule of arriving first is something I'm normally very good at abiding by. But not today. Events in my personal life are taking up much of my time and headspace. Last night, my younger brother was stabbed and robbed in south-west London. He was taken to a local hospital and the family rushed to see him. To our enormous relief, his wound is just a graze and not life threatening. But, while hospital staff are trying to persuade him to stay and receive the treatment he needs, he is keen to discharge himself. For now, he is still in their care, but I know that could change at any time. The situation is weighing heavily on my mind, and this morning I have stumbled blindly through my Underground journey, my thoughts lurching between my brother and Lori.

The professional code for therapists and nurses requires us to leave the personal challenges in our own lives outside the consulting room and to allow our clients to be the priority, giving them space and ensuring that we focus on them. And rightly so. But, for Black therapists, our lived experiences are often very different from those of the white middle-class therapists who dominate the field. We are a part of the very communities that we serve. We're not merely stepping into them from time to time, as an observer might do, viewing things from a distance and then retreating back to our comfortable lives at the end of each day. Too often, we are nursing our own families and friends.

Too often, the violence that we come across in our professional lives is far too close to home.

Ahead of me, a woman holding a large Starbucks coffee spills a little on a man's pricey-looking suit, and he is not impressed. I pass hurriedly between them as she offers a thousand apologies, which will never be enough. Finally, I board my Victoria Line train and wait as patiently as I can while the Tube driver tries to close the doors, all the while asking for a rucksack or a foot to be moved out of the way so that the Tube doors can securely close. 'Mind the gap between the train and platform,' a recorded voice repeatedly says in a London accent. The clock is ticking and this thirty-second hold-up feels like an eternity. I'm painfully aware that it's already ten minutes past nine, and soon Lori will be settling in at the cafe we've selected, coffee in hand, undoubtedly wearing her usual black attire and flicking through her phone, waiting for me. I'm thankful that she's wonderfully calm – a trait I've appreciated in the sessions we've already had. But today is a big day. We're going to talk in detail about the sexual assault she suffered a few months ago and how its lingering aftermath has affected her trust and confidence in the adults around her. That she's ready to open up to me is a testament to her maturity and her self-command. I have to remind myself that Lori is only sixteen years old.

There are no available seats on the Victoria Line train and, as the doors finally close and we move off, I realize I am too short to reach the handrail above my head in order to steady myself. I am unceremoniously flung backwards and only at the last moment do I manage to grab a pole to right myself. I have made quite a bit of noise, and something of a spectacle, and a gentle tap on my hand leads my gaze to a young man of colour who is offering me his seat. I humbly accept his kindness and express my deepest gratitude to him. Such considerate acts from young Black boys are often insufficiently validated. Few people are aware that the polite and respectful side of these young men exists. It needs to be acknowledged, because our societal perception of Black boys allows for only one narrative: that they are badly mannered, dangerous, most probably drug dealers and to be avoided at all costs. I see them more clearly than most and this young man has my full attention as I thank him.

From the comfort of the seat I've been given, I tap out a text to Lori to let her know I am running fifteen or twenty minutes late, but of course there is no phone signal underground, and I begin to worry that she won't wait for me. She is reliable and compliant, and keen to heal herself, but even a nice girl like Lori has other places she needs to be. When I finally tap my travel card to exit at Victoria Station, I see that the text to Lori has been registered as sent. She immediately texts back with 'See you soon' and adds a smiley face for good measure.

As I make my way out to the street, I am reminded of a bloody murder that happened on this spot some years before I started my role with the Gangs Unit. Right here, during the evening rush hour, a group of young people from west London had chased a boy from another school into a corner. In a frenzied attack, they stabbed him multiple times, kicking and punching him to death as he lay on the floor. The case was well covered in the media and the horror of it ripped through the city. In an additional layer to the story, an eighteen-year-old girl – someone not unlike Lori – had been used to buy the knives. It was then that the nurse in me had begun to explore the role that young women play in gang culture. I discovered that what's known as 'honey trapping' is common, where girls are used by men to lure someone to a scene or facilitate a crime. The girls are drawn in by gifts, by flattering words, by something which they hope might be love, only to find themselves stuck. At this point, when there's no way back, they can be used either to buy or to hide a weapon.

When I first received Lori's referral, I was worried that she might have been used as a honey trap by some young men in her circle, but, the more I got to know her, the further my thinking moved away from that possibility. She is vulnerable, certainly, but she is also incredibly bright and analytical; it appears the sexual assault took her by surprise. It has been an unimaginable trauma for her. And trauma, if not addressed, can lead to more trauma and more violence. In the absence of robust therapy and support, reckless, risky and impulsive behaviours can emerge. But this doesn't seem to be the case with Lori. She knows who she is and what she wants to be.

*

Our second session took longer to arrange, as Lori was unexpectedly hesitant in her replies to my text messages. I had to tread carefully. When she eventually agreed to meet, she asked for it to be at my office rather than in a cafe, and she was insistent on this because she wanted to bring along her mother, Tasha. It was Lori's uncertainty about having her mother present that had caused her to procrastinate.

Tasha is still only in her early thirties, a young woman herself; she had Lori when she was just sixteen. I got the impression that Lori wanted to use the therapy session as an opportunity to be honest with her mum for the first time about her feelings. To have someone else in the room with her, a professional who was able to make the space safe, mediate and validate feelings. The idea was that this would allow Lori to express herself to a mother who, I already knew from Lori, was hurting too. Knowing how difficult their relationship had become, I prepared well for the session.

I have experience of working with complex families using a psycho-dynamic and holistic approach to child development and family therapy. I've been involved in cases where children are on the verge of being removed from their parents, and others where they are being reunited with their family after a period of separation. Many of the cases have required the involvement of the courts, with the law, safeguarding, education and health components intersecting. The experience has equipped me with dynamic conflict-resolution tools that promote reflection and growth within families, even when the odds are stacked against them. I could now apply some of these skills to Lori and Tasha. I needed to work out how to facilitate a dialogue between them in a way that ensured a safe space in which feelings could be disclosed. I had faith that Lori could manage the discussion well, but I was less optimistic about her mother's ability to do the same. Despite being so well equipped, I was still slightly anxious about meeting Lori's mum, knowing that I would need to manage some potentially explosive emotions. As it turned out, I wasn't wrong.

On arrival, Tasha made a scene at the clinic reception; she thought one of the receptionists had been off with her. I had to dash downstairs to rescue the situation. I was struck immediately by her wild weave, long painted fingernails, her tight jeans and crop top – she was almost young enough to be one of my patients herself, and certainly looked like one of them. I guided mother and daughter into the meeting room with some placatory words. Tasha tucked herself away in a corner, arms folded tightly and aggressively across her chest. Lori looked defeated already. It was a bad start.

My first task was to try to defuse the atmosphere. I moved around the room carefully, tiptoeing on imaginary eggshells, my eyes firmly on Tasha, then moving to Lori, very purposefully including them both, smiling away, as the British do so well, even when they are at their most uncomfortable. With us all seated, and with a water glass for each of us, I formally thanked Tasha for coming along to the session. She didn't directly acknowledge the gratitude, and I understand now that she didn't want to come across as vulnerable. Instead, she replied by asking me where I am from. Familiar with this loaded question, I made a peace offering of my background and my experience: I told her that I am an African nurse, that I am used to working with young people and communities from our backgrounds, especially those who are troubled. She seemed to relax a little at that, but I knew I didn't necessarily have her with me for long. This was all too painful for her.

I only had some basic knowledge about Tasha's background. While I didn't know for sure if she too had been exposed to sexual exploitation at a young age, my hypothesis was that she very likely had been, and that this might have explained her own teenage pregnancy, her feelings about which she now seemed to be projecting onto her daughter. Either way, I knew that this session would open up old wounds that Tasha would rather remained closed. It was all far too confrontational for her. But Lori needed it to happen. With all this collective trauma, and inherited trauma, Lori needed Tasha to hear what she had to say.

Tasha did not appear to have received any therapy following her childhood experiences. She'd spent the past sixteen years of motherhood coping in the only way she knew, often through passive aggression, and over the past six months had displayed undisguised envy for her daughter. She could see Lori trying to get to grips with her own problems and, against the odds, succeeding, and this had made her uncomfortable. There was a real risk that Tasha could try to sabotage Lori's progress. My job as a therapist was to provide a psychological safe space to allow them both to vent their feelings. But, five minutes into the meeting, I was holding on by a thread.

From nowhere, Tasha blurted out, 'I found used condoms in Lori's bed when she was fifteen. Why was she having sex at fifteen and a half years old? What if she got pregnant? What if she caught something?'

Lori became uneasy, shifting in her chair. Her eyes refused to meet mine. She hadn't revealed to me in our initial session that she had been sexually active before the assault. I was surprised to hear it now, though not shocked. I had to trust that Lori intended to share this with me in her own time and on her terms.

Recovering quickly from her discomfort, Lori stepped in, saying in a low but firm voice, 'Mum, we do not need to keep repeating this. I've apologized several times.'

I felt the need to say something at this point, but Tasha was too fast for me.

'You can't trust these boys, you know,' she said, raising her voice enough to prompt the receptionist to look through the meeting-room window and check that we were all fine. Tasha was getting fully into her stride, out of her seat and spitting her words as she jabbed an angry finger at her daughter. 'The moment you start sleeping with boys, you become a whole woman.'

What Tasha was saying to her daughter, and the defensiveness with which she was saying it, reflected the negativity she had long carried with her about her own actions at Lori's age. I wondered if she was simply trying to communicate her fears for her daughter – that she loves her and wants her to be safe. Perhaps she was trying to say to Lori, *I am terrified that you're going to fall pregnant, just like I did at fifteen. And I am scared that you will mess up your future, like I did.* But volatility and hostility were the only tools at her disposal. She didn't know how to convey her strong emotions differently or better.

Nodding my head in validation of her words, I signalled with an open palm for Tasha to return to her seat. She slowly responded to the request and, with a deep sigh, sat down. I knew she smoked cannabis regularly to cope with life's stresses and I suspected she might have had a joint before coming to the session, to keep the nerves at bay, but she was still volatile. She fidgeted in her seat and kissed her teeth, drawing out the sound in a way that told me loud and clear that she was at the very end of her tether.

Before I could speak, she was off again: 'I told Lori a long time ago not to go to parties she doesn't know anything about, that anything can happen in these places. Now look what has happened.' She threw her hands into the air, as though fire and brimstone were visible to her.

I wanted Tasha to pause, to stop and think through her stinging words before any more came tumbling out, to recognize how damaging they were, that what she says as a mother can cut deeper than the sexual assault itself. I knew she was projecting, that she saw herself in Lori, but she wasn't emotionally equipped to build an attachment with her daughter, let alone support her through this. At the heart of good parenting is the ability to allow the child to grow, the capacity to simultaneously contain a child within safe boundaries and give them the space to explore, to make mistakes and learn from them. Children and adolescents look to their parents for validation, acceptance and safety, but Lori doesn't have these emotional comforts at her disposal. She is going to have to figure out life almost entirely on her own. As her therapist, it is my job to support her while she looks for a positive trajectory into her future, but her background, her past, will never completely leave her be. She will need to learn to coexist with it.

Of the two young women, it was Lori who was demonstrating the greater level of maturity, which suggested to me that she would be able to use our sessions more successfully on her own, and that she would, in time, with a little help, be able to heal herself. She can't control her mother's feelings, and the weight of those emotions are destructive. Without Tasha doing some deep therapeutic work of her own, that isn't going to change. It is a painful but essential conclusion, which Lori has to reach.

The session continued like a boxing match, with Lori attempting to convince her mother that she was trying to make good judgements, but that sometimes she too made mistakes, and with Tasha resisting any opportunity to listen. She refused to validate her daughter's feelings, to say that she was hearing her, that she understood. So, when Tasha stormed out mid-session, I have to admit I was relieved to have time alone with Lori, to allow us both to reflect on what had just happened, and to ensure that, despite all the rage, Lori was feeling safe. In my experience, self-harm is not unusual in victims of sexual assault, and that risk can increase where there's self-blame or lingering guilt. I wanted to remind Lori how incredibly brave she is and that I am here for her, even if her mother isn't.

*

I am well and truly late for today's third session with Lori, and I know I have to compose myself before walking in. The space belongs to her and it is her time to talk, not mine. I don't want my personal challenges to bleed into Lori's; it's inappropriate. The last thing she needs is a frazzled therapist caught up in her own stuff. But, as I leave the station, I can't help but check my phone again. My brother has texted to say that he has discharged himself from hospital. He is heading home and tells me that he will be fine. 'Fine' seems optimistic, but I have to accept defeat and, for now, close that chapter. There is nothing more I can do for him at the moment, but the circumstances of his stabbing linger in my mind.

I walk into the large Pret A Manger off Victoria Street and scan the light-filled room, eventually catching sight of Lori sitting at a small table at the far end. Her head is down. She seems to be flicking through her journal, which she marks up in a coded language that is comprehensible only to her. It's a good way to ensure confidentiality, to protect her innermost thoughts from any prying eyes, including mine.

She senses my arrival and looks up as I approach. I launch in, offering profuse apologies for running late, alluding only to

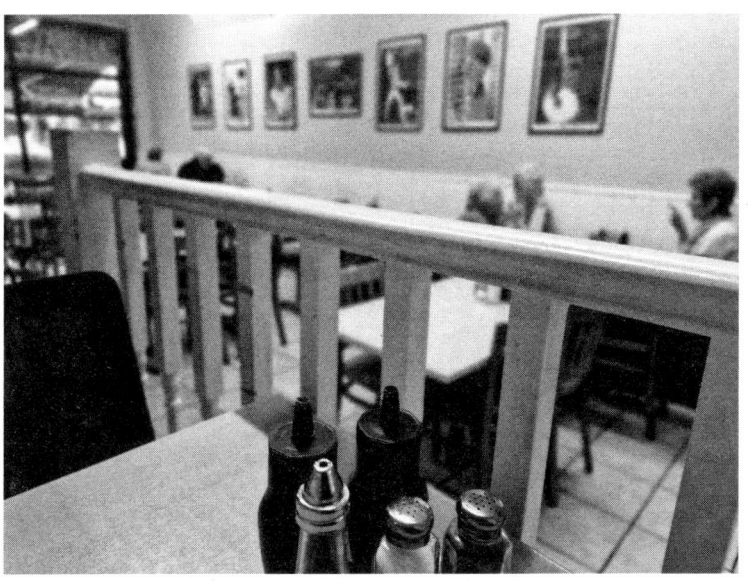

'family challenges' as the cause rather than going into any of the grim detail. But she's at ease with it all. She shrugs her shoulders and smiles up at me.

'Don't worry about it,' she tells me, making space for me to sit down. 'I am used to family chaos.'

We both smile at this as I sit down opposite her, settling into our session.

First, some mindfulness techniques. I ask Lori to reflect on the week that has passed since the meeting with Tasha and to focus on one thing she feels has gone really well in that time. She tells me that she particularly loved a walk she had in Hyde Park, the smell of the cut grass and sight of the pockets of well-tended flowers. I ask her to focus on these two things as we take deep breaths together, synchronizing our breathing, digging deep in the search for calm. We breathe peace into our troubled lives. And, at the end of this shared moment, we look each other in the eye and seal our trust and connection.

In this session, Lori wants to tell me more about the sexual assault, but first needs to address her relationship with her mother, as it has such a bearing on her sense of self and her ability to trust others. She tells me that, since we all met, so unsuccessfully, she has managed to get her mother to talk about the circumstances of her birth. Tasha had struggled with the conversation, crying through most of it. She begged Lori not to walk the same path as she had and talked openly about how those years as a young mother had left her confused and emotionally isolated.

Tasha had nursed Lori, as far as a streetwise sixteen-year-old was able, breastfeeding her for some months, but then she seemed to detach from her daughter, as though the streets were calling her back. She was young; maternity and domesticity were not what she wanted for herself. Tasha went back to her friends and to the parties, leaving Ms Lori to look after her granddaughter. As Lori grew up with her grandmother, Tasha came and went like any other teenager, without a care in the world. Ms Lori was a constant presence, someone with whom Lori still identifies strongly, even though they are a generation apart and culturally adrift.

Lori is still processing this conversation about how she was raised, understanding for the first time just how absent Tasha had been when she was small. It's only since the sexual assault that Tasha has resurfaced as a greater presence in Lori's life, seemingly in order to preach to her daughter about the dangers that lurk after dark in the city, rather than to offer her emotional support. But Lori feels that her mother lost the moral high ground by abandoning her caregiving responsibilities to Ms Lori. Who is Tasha, Lori wonders, to talk to her about men and sex, when Tasha was sexually active herself from the age of fifteen? Although Tasha has finally opened up to her daughter about becoming a mother, and it's clear she wants a closer relationship with Lori, she doesn't know how to go about it. And Lori is afraid of being abandoned again. She can't trust her mother. As a result, each conversation all too easily blows up and gets out of control.

I pause to consult the 'Mood and Feelings' questionnaire that we use in clinic to measure young people's mental health. Unlike most other young people I work with, Lori has been receptive to filling in the forms and texting me the results, demonstrating maturity and taking ownership of her personal development. Since our last meeting, she has filled out a 'Depression and Anxiety' questionnaire and an 'Impact of Events' questionnaire for me. Her responses reveal that she still has more work to do around lessening feelings of guilt and improving her mood. She's still experiencing bouts of anger and some moments of deep sadness, which can be indicative of depression. Depression in young people who have grown up with poor emotional attachments manifests in different ways. Some adolescents take to drug use, some turn to inappropriately sexualized behaviours; violence is not uncommon, nor is complete withdrawal from family and society as a whole. The questionnaire findings are consistent with Lori's presentation today; she's in a relatively good place. But each day brings with it new challenges. How she felt yesterday may be different from how she feels today, or how she may wake up feeling tomorrow. While we are working towards her feeling more consistently positive and in control of her emotions, we still have some way to go.

I ask Lori what she would like to say to her mum if they had a better relationship and were able to be honest with each other, without anger bubbling up and spilling over. She tells me she would like to tell Tasha everything about the assault, how it has left her traumatized, unable to sleep or eat, how she has revisited that night again and again in her mind with deep regret. But she is doubtful that her mother would understand the context in which the assault happened, that Lori hadn't put herself unduly at risk. If her mother would just listen, without comment and without judgement, Lori would like to tell her that, on the night of the assault, she had done all she could to judge the situation, and that, with all she knew about the company she was keeping, she had deemed herself safe. Sitting with me now, she tells me the full story.

*

Lori had been dating Troy for some time. When he suggested they go to a party in a flat in east London, Lori thought nothing of it. There would be a few drinks and they'd be able to hang out with other friends – both things she enjoyed. At the height of the party, in a crowded house that she had never been to before, Troy told Lori that he would be back soon, that he was just picking up 'a little something' from a friend who lived nearby. Again, Lori wasn't concerned, even though her own friends had just left too. She tells me she remembers being tipsy and excited to be somewhere new, intoxicated both by alcohol and the sea of unfamiliar but friendly faces. She remembers speaking to a young man who seemed more sober than everyone else, and registered that he seemed a bit older than her. She remembers talking to him and following him into another room, where he raped her.

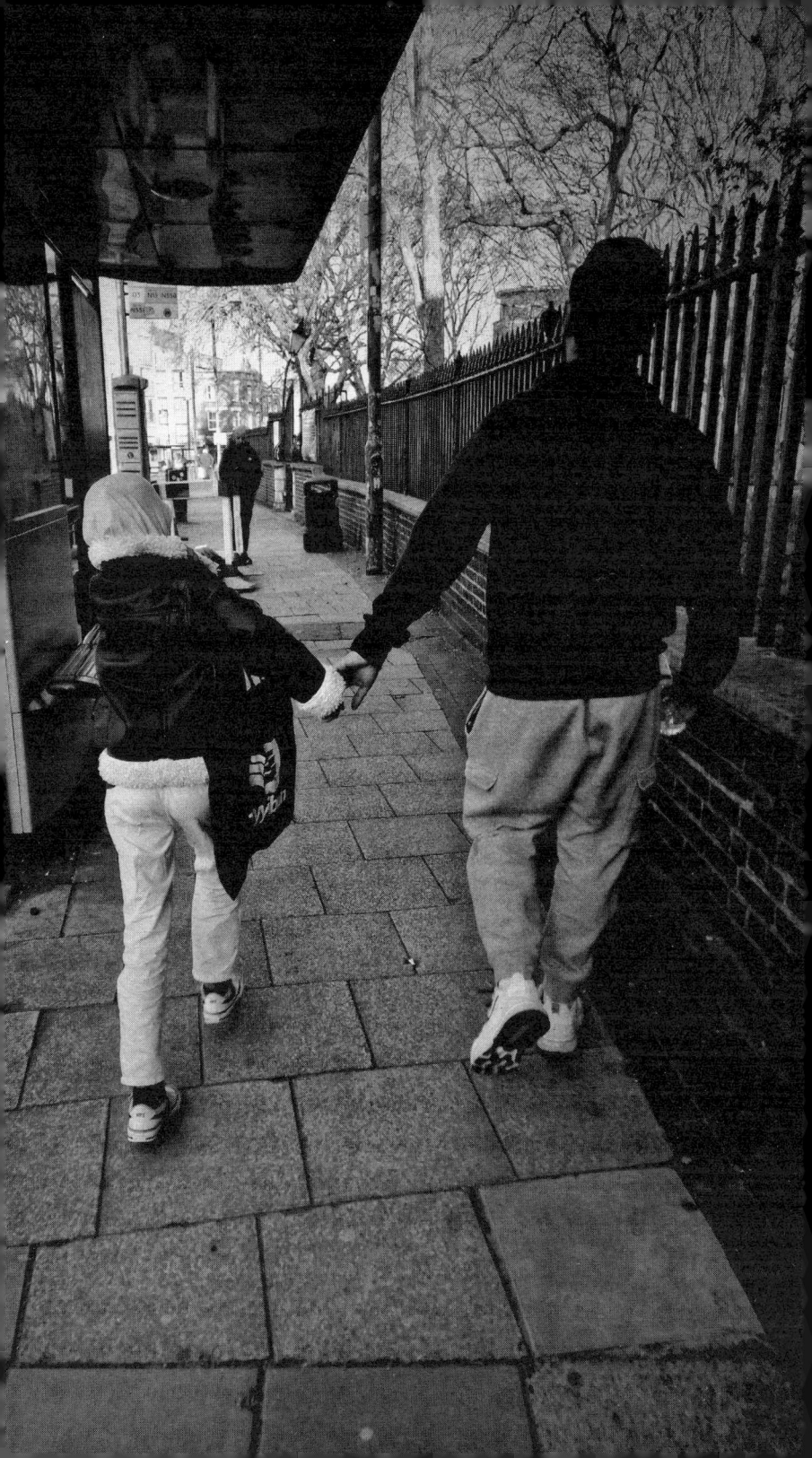

Reeling from what had just happened, she remembers looking around for Troy, calling him and texting him; he hadn't yet returned to the flat. The party was dying down, more people were leaving, and Lori felt alone and desperately wanted to get home. It would take a few night buses, but she began the journey by herself. At some point, Troy eventually picked up his phone, angry at her for leaving the party without him. She in turn blamed him for leaving her alone at a party where she was a stranger, for prioritizing his friends and leaving her vulnerable. She told Troy about the older boy and what had happened in that room. She could hear Troy seething, his anger not directed at the young man who had violated her but at Lori for being alone with him. And his concern was for his own reputation rather than for Lori's safety.

'I know those guys. They were doing it because I left the party,' he said. 'Them guys are just trying to send a message to me, that they can touch you anyhow in my absence.'

Lori and Troy had argued on the phone and had not spoken since. Six months had passed.

She had reported the crime to the police the next day, but had withdrawn her statement soon after for fear there might be reprisals from the assailant and because she realized that she didn't have the strength to see the case through. And she certainly didn't have Troy's support. Feeling defeated when you're at your most vulnerable and barely able to put one foot in front of the other is a common enough feeling among women who have been assaulted. Our national statistics on sexual assaults are grim. Rape Crisis England and Wales reports that fewer than 3 per cent of rape cases recorded by the police result in someone being charged for the offence, let alone convicted. And these are just the cases that are reported. Most victims don't follow through, and, for those who do, some may face a wait of as long as two years before the case comes to court.

Our services weren't there to support Lori. And neither was her mum.

Since the assault, Lori's mood has been down. She has self-harmed, and thoughts about hurting herself further are bothering her. They're bothering me, too. To help her in her search for answers as to why this happened to her and how she can move forward, I asked her to draft a letter to her mother, and she has brought it with her to the session today. She hands a neatly handwritten page to me.

The letter is an outpouring of grief about what Lori calls *a life full of stains*: of fighting, of rape, of not knowing who her father is. Lori tells her mother that she wants to wash these stains away, and is using therapy to help her, but that all she really wants is a hug from her mother. *You had me at sixteen. I'm sixteen now and I've been raped*, she tells her. *I know this scares you. It scares me too, but I want us to do this healing journey together. We both need to heal from so much. Mum, I am aching. I am worn out. I am tired of my own tears.* Lori tells her mother that the grudges they hold against each other are wearing her down. While Tasha is angry with Lori for having sex at fifteen, she is frustrated that Tasha can't see the condoms as evidence of her trying to protect herself. *I am trying to grow up as best as I can*, she writes. *Mum—*

And there the words stop. I flip the page over. There's nothing. Lori has come as far as she can. What she doesn't dare to write down is that, despite the terrible setback she has experienced, she is on her way to exercising her freedom and growing into a confident young woman – an unimaginable dream in Tasha's world. Despite what has happened to her, Lori will have everything that Tasha might have once aspired to, but hasn't achieved. Lori has structure in her life. She has emotional intelligence. She has hope. She is clear about who she is. She knows she can use this to carve out a pathway to healing. Tasha didn't have these qualities as a teenager and still lacks them now as a mother, in which role she is expected to support her daughter. Instead, she has set out to make Lori's life as difficult as possible. Across the table, Lori looks back at me steadily, and I see that, for her, there are fewer questions about how to make everything right with her mother. Right now, she's simply in search of the hug that has never been on offer.

I see that Lori is fighting hard to hold back the tears. She rolls her shoulders, straightens up, breathes deeply, in through her nose and out through her mouth, trying to drive them away. But the flood can't be stemmed. Tears spill over and black mascara streaks down her cheeks. She continues to look at me, making no effort to wipe them away. In this moment, she is exposed and raw, a young woman who has fallen into a deep hole of sorrow and is struggling to lift herself out of an emotional mess that is not of her making. She fights to compose herself, finally wiping her eyes and face carefully with her fingertips. I reach out and touch her hand, then I squeeze tight and feel it tremble beneath mine.

'Oh, but you are so strong, Lori – stronger than you know,' I say to her.

'I'm not. I look like I'm strong, but the truth is sometimes it's hard.' She shakes her head, her voice reduced to a whisper: 'Really hard.'

'I know that,' I reply. 'But I see you using these experiences to better your life, to break the cycle and to create your own narrative.'

'Sometimes it's just too hard, but I keep trying,' she says, allowing more tears to wash down her cheeks. If only they could wash away her troubles.

As the tears finally subside, she carefully wipes her face again and tries once more to compose herself, taking a few deep breaths in a moment of mindfulness, and this time succeeding.

I smile as I watch her. It's a coping mechanism that I've shared with her and it has had a huge impact on her ability to manage her emotions. She's growing as an individual right in front of my eyes.

'You will be fine, Lori,' I whisper to her, smiling into her lovely face. And I think she believes that she will.

*

As I make my way back to Victoria Station, my mind stays on Lori. She is realizing that she can't change the way people around her think and act, but she can change herself. She has control over her own life and, although she doesn't have the support of her mother, there is love and warmth in her life. She has friends. She has her grandmother. She'll continue to have therapy and she will keep developing her coping mechanisms, using mindfulness and journalling to deal with her stress. She is learning how and who to trust; she will keep her distance from Troy and the young man who raped her. And she is working on self-protection, not allowing herself to be drawn into situations that might pose a risk to her safety.

Tasha, I know, needs her own therapy to address the issues that are wearing her down and preventing her from being close to her daughter, but it won't be me who's able to help her – it's beyond the scope of my work. In any case, she isn't ready yet. But I am hopeful that the time will come.

Outside the station, I allow myself a last moment to think about Lori and our work together, and to celebrate how far she has come. It's this that gives me the strength to find my phone and make a call to my brother.

'It's me,' I say when he picks up. 'How are you?'

4. Amir: The Mosque

> *'When it comes to socio-economic disadvantage, children from these families are at higher risk of autism – but having a child with autism can also increase the risk of poverty.'*

THE THIRTY-MINUTE WALK along the canal, carved out of the earth between the bustling market and the majestic mosque, offers the chance for a moment of reflection. Today, this pause for contemplation feels more necessary and restorative than ever. At the best of times, I find crisp autumn walks soothing. Walking always clears my head, offering as it does a rare and sacred moment of solitary silence, a peace that's hard to come by in my day-to-day life. But today is the worst of times. I am readying myself to step into the mosque's women's quarter for Amir's funeral. Each footstep in the fresh air is tonic preparing me for the challenges that lie ahead. The elegant city geese gliding along the canal and the affluent homes that back onto it are a welcome distraction.

Today, I need to tap into the highest version of myself, the professional nursing persona which I trust will guide me through the events of the next few hours. I need to think carefully about how I will behave, what I will say, how I will listen and how I might help. Amir was stabbed outside the school gates on the very last day of the school year. And, today, his family and friends are gathering together to remember him and to offer their prayers. There is nothing in all the hours of nursing training that prepares you for the death of a teenager. There's

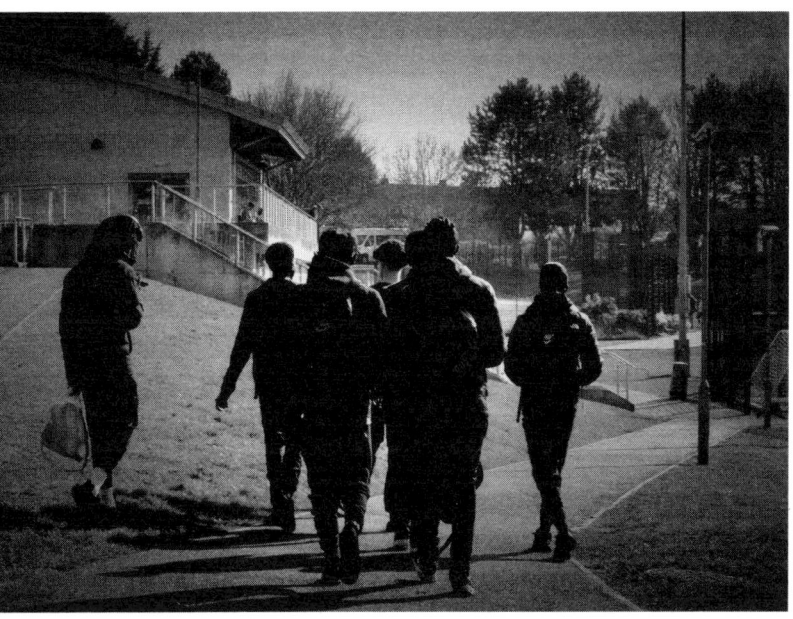

even less guidance for how you might deal with that child being stabbed in the same streets that you walk daily and on which you choose to nurse your patients. I am on uncertain ground. I am feeling my way.

The past few months have felt unusually long. The heatwave we've experienced in London has been like the full force of Mother Nature's anger, so incandescent with rage that she has

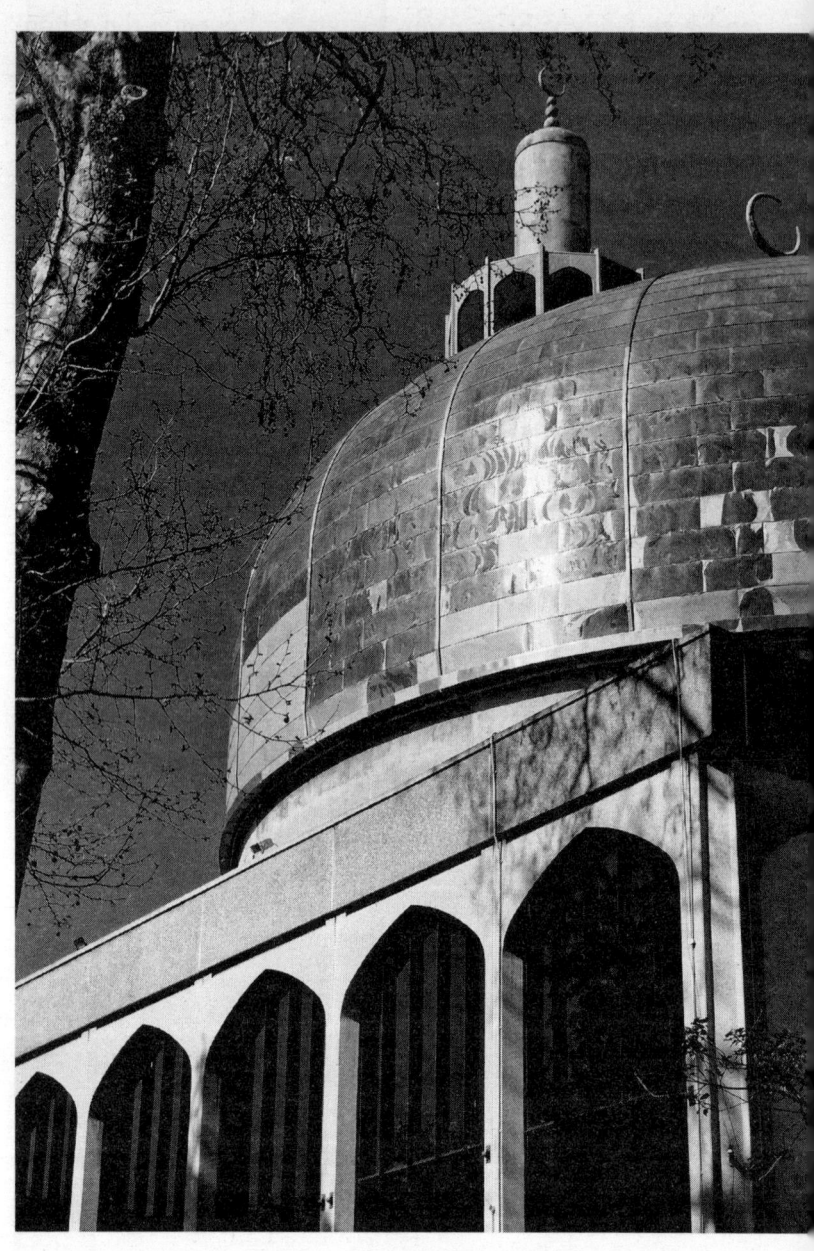

set fire to fields and woodland and to homes. She has dried up the reservoirs and scorched the earth. Activists have had to remind us, yet again, just how much we have neglected our future. It's a message that screams all the louder on a day when a child is being buried.

This part of London is an area that has experienced rapid gentrification. In addition to the carefully plotted period mansions and densely packed council housing, the past few years have seen the erection of spectacular apartments and modern offices, as well as the proliferation of trendy coffee houses. Well-kept barge homes line the canal, a lifestyle choice. The Turkish food stall that used to sell fresh fruit and vegetables has been bested by a Starbucks and a Pret A Manger, both doing excellent business. The local chip shop is long gone, so too the greasy spoon. Cranes pepper the skyline – there is more development to come. I've seen the change happening bit by bit, then all of a sudden, because I have walked this route many times to nurse my patients in my street clinic. But never before to bury one.

A parent should never have to bury their child, I think, as I walk along the canal. But in a world full of violence and anger, hatred and ignorance, today Nour is saying goodbye to her son. She has asked me to support her at the mosque. It's an unusual nursing intervention, and I am honoured to spend the afternoon at her side. Knowing all about her poor health, I have already reminded Nour not to forget her hypertension tablets and to keep an eye on her blood sugars throughout the day. But my primary concern is her mental well-being. Amir was Nour's only son. How does a mother cope with the death of her only son?

Nour's request for me to support her today shows the trust that has grown between us since that first hesitant meeting; she recognizes the deep respect I feel for her and the value she places on family and her faith. But, while I am honoured, the enormity of the occasion threatens to overwhelm me. I am working hard to portray a calm and professional exterior, an impression of complete control, but my legs are trembling. I am anxious. I remember what my mentors and supervisors have always told me: that it is safer to be nervous than to be overconfident and complacent. I decide that perhaps I am exactly as I should be: full of compassion and ready to help in any way I can.

*

It has been a dramatic eight months since Amir was urgently referred to me through my work in the Gangs Unit. Amir's was a case that had slipped through the net. He had been allocated a social worker, but at some point his case had been closed by social services. Getting the young person and their family to engage is the core challenge for all bodies concerned, including the Gangs Unit. Things had been further complicated by Amir's mother being reluctant to speak to the school and other services; she was wary of them. Besides, there was a language barrier and, every time she needed to speak to someone, her daughter, Nadia, would have to take time off work to support her, so Nour found it easier to retreat. Before the Gangs Unit came on board, all the talk had got her nowhere.

When all was said and done, few professionals were willing to see Amir for the vulnerable child he was. The hope was that the Gangs Unit could support Amir, and help to keep him safe and out of gangs. Although a clear autism diagnosis had never been made because of the family's migratory history and patchy healthcare records, he was showing signs of challenging behaviours: oppositional, impulsive, angry. When we first met him, he had been involved in petty crime and a number of fights, in the streets and inside school, and he was on the verge of exclusion from mainstream education, facing a new environment at a Pupil Referral Unit.

The referral notes indicated that he came from a single-parent home, that his mother, a consistent presence in his life, had a number of health problems of her own, including high blood pressure, diabetes and stress. Additionally, the family had missed a number of mainstream clinic appointments and was now deemed 'hard to reach'. Given my experience as a mental-health practitioner and my additional skills in safeguarding vulnerable groups, as well as my experience in working with excluded or marginalized families, I was asked to work with Amir and, by extension, his mother too. The hope was that I could engage them and lessen their mental-health burden. By connecting with them, I might be able to reduce some of the risks and improve their health outcomes.

A referral of this kind identifies the young person as the main focus of our work, but we all recognize the difficulties young people can have engaging with professionals, so, where appropriate, we also work with the wider family, building trust and developing psychological safety. It's a dynamic that has been mastered by the team's youth workers. When I first spoke to Amir over the phone, with his youth worker Stephen on the call too, he wasn't terribly receptive, but I persisted in the hope that we could help not just Amir but his whole family to turn things around.

Stephen and I had arranged a joint home visit, and I met him outside the block of flats where Amir lived. Stephen had started out as an assistant support worker in community centres, moving across into the field of youth work later. And he was good at it. He had been working with Amir for some time, so he knew the family well. He had a good relationship with them, which we could leverage. He was also familiar with the neighbourhood; he had a solid understanding of all the children and families who were at risk in Amir's area. And there were a lot of them.

Our visit to the family home was organized through Amir's

older sister, Nadia. Nadia was just twenty-one years old, but I learned from Stephen that she was the one who coordinated all the family's health appointments and tried to ensure that her mother and brother turned up to them. She didn't always succeed. She had taken time off from her internship in a law firm to meet with us, keen to ensure that all the strings tied together and that her brother got the help he needed. It was a lot of responsibility placed on very young shoulders.

We made our way to the family's two-bedroom flat on the upper floor of one of the estate's low-slung houses, which were dwarfed by the surrounding high-rises. As we approached, I recognized Amir standing on the walkway. He was impressively tall and slim, with a wonderfully youthful face. I could see his arms waving in the air as he talked, his legs in constant motion. He was surrounded by a group of school-age people, all chatting and talking over each other.

'Bruv, it ain't even like that . . .' I heard Amir say.

'Innit, innit, innit . . .' a chorus of teenagers seemed to echo.

I momentarily locked eyes with Amir, and he quickly looked away. I knew better than to try to engage with him while he was in the middle of performing this bravado. This was his time, and we were on his territory. Right now, his friends mattered most. I knew that I had a better chance of speaking with him in his home environment – or perhaps in his school – than here on the street, so I kept up my pace and carried on walking, following closely in Stephen's footsteps. He too knew the game. We could only hope that, at some point, Amir would join us.

The front door of the flat was open; Nadia and her mother Nour were expecting us.

Confident and knowledgeable, Nadia led the conversation. After introducing us to Nour, she dived straight into the issues, her eyes focused on the familiar Stephen. But Nour was looking at me intensely. I knew that, like most of the wary mothers

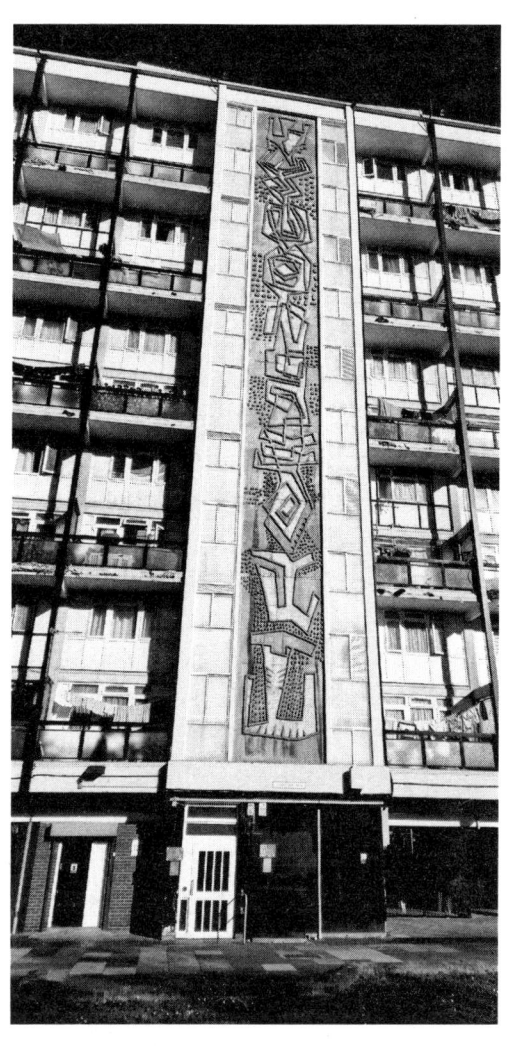

I had encountered, she was trying to place me culturally before she could begin to trust me.

'From Nigeria?' she asked, speaking across her daughter.

'Zimbabwe,' I replied with a smile.

I already knew that Nour had been born in a small village in Algeria, and that Amir had been born in France. She nodded.

It's not unusual for the parents I work with to be inquisitive about the backgrounds of the people who have been put in place to support them, particularly those who feel they have been let down by the NHS and the other services. Some families are reluctant to engage with professionals from a white background, especially if they've had prior experience of racism or discrimination. This means some have a preference for youth workers or medical professionals from minority backgrounds. And, perhaps, in terms of being fully understood, they have a point. For most, religion tends to be less of an issue, not least because Britain has become such a secular society. But the question of whether the worker has their own children or not comes up often. With these loaded preconceptions in mind, I knew I had more work to do to settle Nour's anxiety about who I was and what I could offer. Stephen reassured both women, explaining that I was an experienced nurse and that I was well accustomed to working with young people and families from a wide range of backgrounds. Nour nodded again, satisfied – for now, at least.

Balancing compassion and care while bringing the focus back to Nour and her needs, we set about creating a psychological safe space for her to share her experiences. I gently asked Nour about her own health and how the challenges she was facing with Amir might be affecting her – and we began to talk. There is a strong correlation between poor physical health and poor mental health, and this can be exacerbated with poverty. Many of the parents I work with have physical health challenges, such as hypertension, pancreatitis, cancer or physical disability.

Nour was no exception. I asked her how she was coping with her hypertension and diabetes, emphasizing the importance of ensuring she didn't stress excessively over issues that we both knew were extremely stressful.

I encouraged her to take some time away from the house, to sit in the local park enjoying the fresh air, even if only for twenty minutes. I encouraged her to eat and sleep well, knowing how difficult it is to eat and sleep well, let alone leave the house and sit in a park, when your child is involved with gangs. Feeling safe with me, Nour shared how the last few weeks had been tough, how she sometimes felt aches and pains for which she couldn't find a cause. She also felt guilty about leaving it to Nadia to hold the family together, a responsibility that was threatening

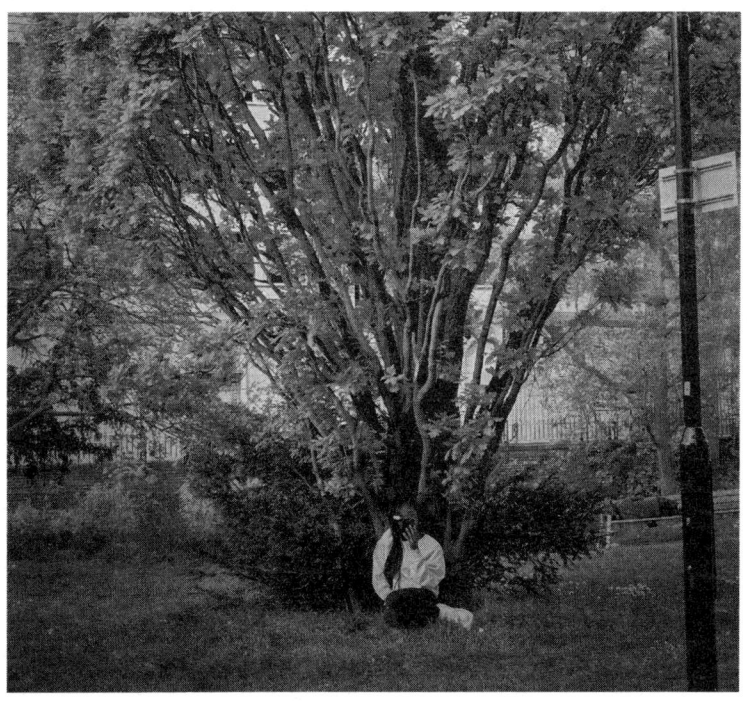

the internship which she'd struggled to secure.

I listened to Nour. I heard her and I felt her pain.

This was the first of several home visits that I would make to Nour, but Amir would try to keep his distance, seeing no real need for help at all, but acknowledging that, if help was to come, it should be directed at his mum. He too was concerned about his mother's health and the impact stress was having on her. His was an indirect way of caring for his poorly parent. But, while many young people like Amir have some idea of the impact of their behaviours on their parents and address it, some do not.

*

The weeks before Amir was stabbed had been intense. The argument – or 'beef', as the kids like to say, but which downplays how serious a disagreement can become – had been building at the Pupil Referral Unit where he had been sent after being excluded from mainstream education. Police and social workers had attended the school on several occasions, and while the health sector was involved too, it wasn't to the extent required, given what was unfolding. Typically, a young person who is excluded from school and placed in a Pupil Referral Unit would have a team of professionals working around them, especially if they have a suspected or confirmed diagnosis of autism.

The team is designed to support the young person's developmental needs, which include health, social and educational needs. The professional bodies might include social services, teachers, nurses, general practitioners, youth workers and community workers. This should be the standard for all vulnerable young people. But, where care is poor or fragmented, some professional bodies become preoccupied with the young person's displays of violence rather than the reasons for it. Their own fears and preconceptions of violence can get in the way of addressing a young person's needs. Although physical risk should never be underestimated, it's important to find a balance between care, enforcement and development.

No one was there to protect Amir and equip him with the skills needed to build some resilience and employ coping mechanisms against the turbulent streets that he had to navigate. His autistic traits increased his vulnerability; his ability to manage his emotions and cope with change was compromised. Autism is a condition that requires support, consistency and regulation for individuals to thrive. In the end, Amir had no one to help him find a better way to cope with his stress than smoking cannabis and using his fists. By the time he was referred to the Gangs Unit, he was already a long way down a criminal pathway and turning back didn't feel like an option.

Pupil Referral Units are, I think, best explained by comparing them to prisons for children. They are where the British education system dumps all of its young people who are excluded from mainstream schools. When the schools can't cope, when a child's behaviour has become too much for the teaching staff, the child is asked to leave. The jury is still out on whether we should be excluding these vulnerable children from education or not, but what we do know is that, once excluded, they become vulnerable to being recruited into gangs. Many of these excluded children have learning difficulties. Some are socially and environmentally predisposed to challenging behaviours, such as bullying, fighting in school or outside in the streets, engaging in impulsive and explosive behaviours that put others at risk, or bringing dangerous weapons into school. Absenteeism in these young people is common and often fostered by parents who should be encouraging their children to go to school and educate themselves out of their situation, if possible. When all of these children who are excluded from mainstream education are put in one place, like a Pupil Referral Unit, it becomes fertile ground for gangs.

Amir had been humiliated on a daily basis in the corridors of the PRU and in its playground. He had been humiliated on social media, with other kids mocking his lingering French accent and mimicking his autistic traits, posting reels for all to see. Nour told me that Amir was particularly hurt because the boy who led the mockery had been his friend. At least, that's what Amir thought. In search of the truth about their relationship, and to find out who was spreading rumours about his autistic traits and saying that girls didn't like him, Amir confronted his friend. The friend recorded the brief encounter to further humiliate Amir on social media. The animosity escalated, and they hissed vicious words and sized each other up as a hungry audience looked on. When the fight broke out in front of the school gates, in broad daylight, right there in full view of the CCTV cameras that would capture everything, Amir would not have known that his 'friend' was carrying a knife.

Schoolchildren, particularly those in a PRU, love watching a fight. They quickly get wind of when one is brewing, through urgent whispers in the school corridors and bathrooms and frantic social-media notifications. Gang members will take their positions, measuring up the situation, debating who will jump whom, and who will instigate the fight. They seem to know who the winners and losers will be even before the fight breaks out, whom to get behind and whom to throw to the wolves. The bystanders – and there will always be bystanders to egg on the participants – are like extras in a film. The scene would feel less real without them. They circle, inviting the weaker opponent into the fray to humiliate themselves further. Once the opponents are both in the fight circle, the spectators close around them, their hands in the air, fists pumping, encouraging the violence. Many will have their phones out; fights are always recorded. Like data, or entertainment, they must be shared and evaluated. The dramatic story is documented for everyone's eyes. And it's a story full of tragedy.

One of the girls looking on is likely to have been used to buy the knife that will shortly be plunged into a teenager's body as easily as slicing a meat loaf. This queen bee is probably dating one of the fighters, who, in her eyes, demonstrates the highest level of masculinity. But too often these girls have no understanding of what true masculinity is. They are likely to have been involved in street fights themselves, with girls from other schools or areas of town. Violence among girls can play out in much the same way, but social media is their primary battleground. And social media is also where fights are instigated, ultimatums are set, and where the results are posted.

Suicides and self-harming behaviours can stem from there.

The link between gang involvement and suicide or self-harm has been explored by American academic Adam Watkins, who published his team's work under the title 'Bad Medicine'. The relationship between gang membership and negative emotional behaviours is very clear. Young people who become involved in gangs are at higher risk of depression and self-harm, and are more likely to decide that life isn't worth living.

The girls shame each other's bodies; they attack each other for being too slim or too short or too fat – the kind of abuse that often leads to eating disorders. For them, posting anything on social media is an act of bravery. It's an act that provokes anxiety. They know that whatever they say can and will be received differently in different circles, wilfully misinterpreted and misunderstood. But surviving fights gives them clout. If the violence moves from social media to real life, then it's likely they will seriously injure someone in a vicious brawl. The victim will probably be hospitalized and certainly traumatized to the point that they are no longer seen on the streets. In a world where anything said or done involves taking a risk, violence speaks. These girls have a reputation for a reason; just like the boys, they are to be feared.

It's the sound of these young girls' hysteria which often draws a bigger crowd to the fight scene, and the insistent chant will begin: 'Beef, beef, beef!' It's then that the teachers finally get wind of the fight, hearing it before they see it. And they come running.

When the fighting ring closed around Amir that afternoon, he was seething, raging, livid. He was armed only with his clenched fists. His heart was pounding and he was breathing hard and fast, his light skin flushed red. Adrenalin rushed through his veins. His lungs filled with oxygen. His brain became more alert, sending signals to his young limbs so that his body mobilized and readied itself. Amir was in fight-or-flight mode, and he chose to fight. The decisions he made in that split second were instinctive, unthinking. And, that afternoon, Amir did not make it out of the ring.

As the knife was inserted into Amir's heart, the CCTV footage shows, his body staggered backwards and fell onto the pavement, blood seeping through his white shirt. The audience of excited schoolchildren quickly dispersed. Teachers rushed in, two or three of them calling the ambulance and the police as they ran. What seemed like moments later, a police helicopter arrived, hovering over the school and the surrounding area, scanning all activity and trying, no doubt, to collect evidence, to spot someone running through the streets. But their arrival was too late for Amir. They had not been there to protect him when he needed them most.

*

Nour told me that she'd heard the helicopter first. She'd been at home, it was an ordinary day, and she'd thought nothing much of it. This is London, after all; there's often a helicopter circling. Her phone had been on charge all afternoon, and on silent. When she eventually picked it up, she saw she had many missed calls from the school and from a few of Amir's friends. It was then that the police knocked on her door. When Nour opened it, she knew immediately that this would be the darkest day of her life.

She told me that, on that last day of school, Amir had been unsure about going in. He had been angry and restless in the days leading up to the incident, checking social media constantly, obsessed by who liked a post and who didn't. He would suck his teeth as he rifled through the contents of the fridge, discontent with everything he found there and turning down his mother's cooking, his appetite lost. He had complained bitterly of a headache several times over the last few days. He hadn't been sleeping much and had used the toilet frequently. He became panicked if he thought he had left his phone somewhere that wasn't within reach. Nour had thought nothing much of it; he was a teenage boy, after all. Things were always happening in his life – so-called 'drama' – that caused upset, and then just as quickly they would pass.

In moments of what Nour would later recognize as desperation, Amir had asked her if his French accent really did stand out, or were the kids at school just exaggerating? She told him that there was absolutely nothing wrong with having been born in France. After all, she had been born in a village in Algeria, and what was so wrong with that? She reminded him that his grandfather had migrated from a rural village in Algeria to France with very little education. He had worked hard and eventually owned a local restaurant on the outskirts of Paris. He had done well. She told Amir that there was much more to him than met the ignorant eye, and that there was life for him beyond the school gates and he should focus on that.

Nadia had been harder on her brother. As he fussed around his food and complained about his head aching, she reminded him how spoilt he was. She repeatedly told him that he wouldn't be in this situation – dreading going to school, uncertain about who his friends were – had he not got himself excluded from mainstream education for smoking cannabis and getting into fights. Nadia blamed their mother for being too lenient with him because he was a boy, pointing out that she was much stricter with her, the girl. When Nour felt cornered by the conflict between her children, her instinct was to protect Amir even more, excusing his smoking and fighting by saying he was 'just trying to be a man'.

Perhaps, I thought, Amir was trying to model what he thought was missing in their lives: a husband and a father. Amir's father was distant, removed from their daily lives. In his absence, it was Nadia who'd assumed the role of breadwinner and disciplinarian. But Nadia was irritated, her emotions running close to the surface, because she always had to pick up the pieces from Amir's fallouts. She had been there when the family tried to negotiate with the mainstream school not to exclude him. She had been there when he was arrested and taken into police custody for the use of drugs. And she was here now, trying to help Amir adjust to the PRU.

At first, when the arguments at school and on social media had begun to escalate, Nour had told Amir not to worry. But, of course, he did. Amir was worried about his image, about whether he fitted in or not, whether he was British or not. He certainly felt more British than French. So, he had skipped a few days of school in the hope that the bullying might ease off – if he was out of sight, perhaps he'd be out of mind. But it didn't seem to help. He thought he had found allyship with one of the bigger boys, but after a while he seemed to reject him too. And rejection was hard. It made Amir feel less than.

He felt excluded, again. It was an emptiness similar to when his father had left and moved back to Paris to live with his other family.

*

Death scares me, even as a nurse, although I should probably be used to it by now. But it also scares me as a member of society, because I see the impact every death has on a community. Each death reminds me of my own long days of grief, when we lost our brothers to HIV/AIDS in Zimbabwe. The virus wreaked havoc through many communities. We buried too many.

Culture and Christianity mingle at African funerals. In our Shona culture, the body is buried around three to four days after death. It is brought back home so that the deceased can sleep at home for the last time. Mourners circle the body in dance and trance throughout the night as the African drums beat. They sing songs of honour – this is a celebration of a life well lived – and pain is expressed by wailing, screaming and rolling on the ground. Grief hangs in the air, and all the while people pass by and say to the bereaved family, '*Nematambudziko*'. Sorry for your loss. Death is dark, and the death of a child is even darker. There are many moments in which to lose yourself in search of meaning and understanding. That search is a global phenomenon. It is not the preserve of a single culture.

In our Shona culture, patriarchy sets the tone for the funeral. The men will make the big decisions, organizing for a body's repatriation, for example, when someone dies in England or elsewhere and the body needs to be taken back to Zimbabwe. And they will decide where the burial will take place, either in the rural area where that person's life began or in the city where they felt at home. But women also play a discreet and powerful role, especially when it comes to the nitty-gritty of proceedings. The matriarchs of the family, or aunties, with their wide hips,

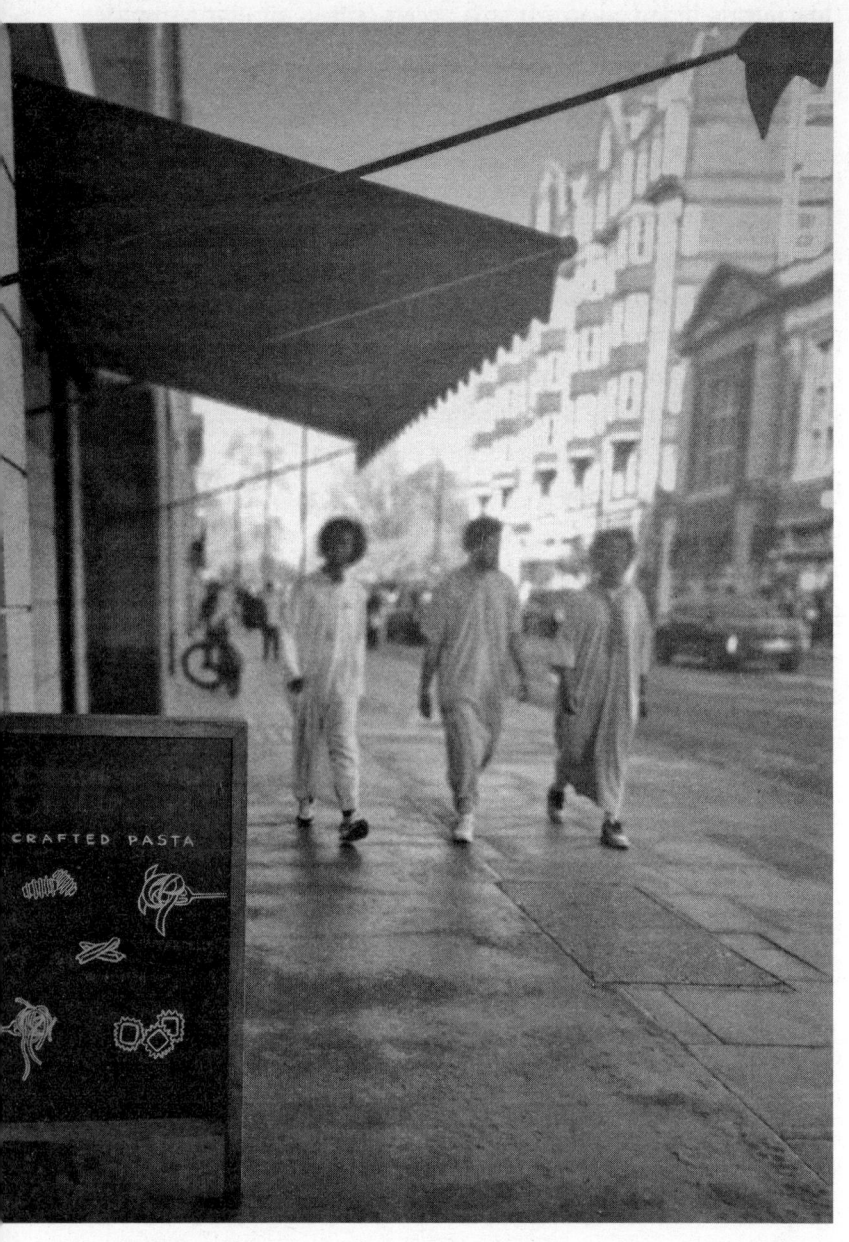

their heads wrapped in colourful scarves, are very visible and sometimes overbearing, as though the grief is theirs alone, and all the men scurry to execute their wishes. Many parental decisions, such as who will take care of the orphans, run through matriarchal channels. Sometimes families will decide that they need to consult traditional healers on the 'real cause of death', a practice upheld by elders but too often looked down upon by the younger generation. But, if the matriarchs decide it should proceed, then proceed it will. These African women are the glue that holds the family together, the silent breadwinners, the constant and the core.

But I am in London, now, and things are done differently here.

*

I exit the canal path onto a wealthy avenue where the impossibly lavish homes may be objectively beautiful, but to me seem soulless. Everyone who lives here is, of course, completely oblivious to the funeral taking place just a stone's throw away. But I want the whole of London to stop, listen and feel the impact of Amir's loss. I want to stand on the tallest building in London and shout at the top of my lungs. I want to remind the city that, if we keep losing our teenagers to senseless knife crime, we will lose a generation. And that isn't right. Why does no one seem to care?

Ahead, I begin to see people: Amir's community. A small crowd has started to fill the road leading to the mosque. Amir's father will be here somewhere, among the mourners. I have never met him, but I know he must be here to bury his son. Stephen will be supporting him and the wider male family. My focus is on Nour and Nadia.

Groups of women move slowly together, their long dresses sweeping the pavement. There are many young people here –

young men who look just like Amir, and young women too. I recognize one or two, but don't approach them to say hello; it doesn't seem appropriate to intrude on their thoughts, the spiritual territory they're occupying today. It's common for young people to attend their friends' funerals, and I'm glad to see this turnout, but some funerals can be tense, volatile, even hostile. Violence can erupt even in the depths of sorrow. But Amir's funeral feels calm and peaceful, as if Amir himself has declared a ceasefire, at least for today.

I adjust my long black skirt, remove my light black jacket from around my waist and slip it back on. I have been intentional about what I'm wearing today. I fussed for hours, knowing that my nursing uniform or hospital scrubs wouldn't be appropriate for Amir's funeral. Today is about nursing within the community, expressing love and friendship, not about the services that Amir and his family accessed. The services that let them down.

I approach the mosque and mingle with the small groups that are milling at the entrance as if trying to delay the moment when Amir will officially be gone from their lives. All the while, I look out for Nour and Nadia.

Eventually, it's time to go inside, and the grand scale of the main mosque is, at first sight, overwhelming. Its pillars stand tall, with worshippers and mourners moving around them purposefully and with deep respect. I follow a stream of young women in elegant hijabs to the female quarter.

A few young men of Middle Eastern origin edge past me as the call to prayer, the azan, sounds through the speakers. I am mesmerized, honouring this holy space. As I listen, I allow myself to drift into a spiritual trance of my own for a moment, swept away by the powerful, deeply soothing sound and its ability to unite people at a time of need.

A soft voice breaks into my thoughts.

'Doci, Doci, are you looking for my mum?'

Like many of my patients, Nadia and Nour have never been able to pronounce my name correctly, so they have adjusted it to what they can work with, and I've made no objection. I choose my battles. More importantly, I need their trust and connection, and nothing is to be achieved by fighting over a name's pronunciation.

Nadia seems collected and contained in her grief. Her brother's murder has taken her out of her internship role, at least for the time being. She is now the sole head of the home and, whether or not it's a role she embraces, she is doing it and doing it well. I can only hope that the crushing weight of Amir's murder on the family does not rob her of her independence.

'Thank you for coming,' Nadia says graciously. She turns away from me for a moment to acknowledge another mourner.

When I have her attention again, I look into her tired eyes, which only now start to brim, and say, 'I am so sorry for your loss.'

She manages a half-smile. 'Doci . . .' she says, for the first time without the words to express herself.

Nadia's friends begin to surround her, young British women, many of whom appear to be of North African descent and some of Middle Eastern origin, all weeping, sobbing and praying. 'Allah,' they repeatedly whisper.

Over their heads, Nadia finds me with her eyes and points me in her mother's direction. She knows that Nour needs support today.

Nadia has been translating for her mother whenever needed and consulting with the wider family in Algeria. They too have had a say in what happens today, although, like everyone else, they were unable to help Amir in that moment when he was stabbed outside the school gates. Their faith and their values have been the constant, helping them through it all. Nothing tests the strength of a family like the death of a loved one abroad.

The Algerian community in London has put its arms around Nour and Nadia. Their response is powerful in so many ways, and yet completely powerless in the face of this vicious knife crime in their own neighbourhood, on their own doorstep.

*

The women's quarter of the mosque is on the balcony of the main prayer room. The staircase leading to it is spotless and the walls clean and bare. In a fountain of bubbling water in the corner, women are busy washing their hands and feet. Other mourners kneel on the prayer room's soft carpet, its soothing red and brown colours reminding me of the rich Iranian rugs that will be found in the surrounding wealthy homes. The room is full, not just with Amir's mourners, but with everyday worshippers who are passing through for prayer and a spiritual moment in an otherwise hectic day. In the midst of the hubbub, I find Nour sitting on a chair, surrounded by other women, elders and relatives. She is inconsolable. I reach out to gently touch her hand, but another hand gets there first. I can't reach her.

'I am the nurse,' I whisper to the small crowd around her.

'Ah, she is the nurse, the nurse, let her come closer,' various voices say.

At a time of grief, the most important intervention that a nurse can offer is a psychological safe space that allows for silence. It is important to be explicitly present. And it is crucial to possess the cultural competency skills which recognize that each person grieves in their own way and at their own pace. The mosque is offering Nour and the other mourners a space of deep spiritual comfort; my intention today is for my nursing interventions to support that.

I lean into Nour, trying to get closer. As she looks up at me and into my eyes, I can see she is hurting. Today is so hard for all of us, but it is hardest for her. It will take some time before she finds any closure. Perhaps she never will.

'I am sorry, Nour.' I whisper in her ear. 'I am so sorry,' I repeat.

I remain close to her, my hand on top of hers, searching for it again when another mourner comes between us. I want to stay as near as possible to her. I notice that her breathing is shallow; she is holding her chest as if she's having trouble breathing. I move closer again and gently ask the mourners to give her some space, to let her breathe with ease. They nod and conform, stepping back.

'Ambulance, shall we call the ambulance?' someone asks.

I look to Nour, who says, 'No ambulance, please. No ambulance.'

What she's communicating to us is that her grief is deep, so deep that it's affecting her breathing, yet there is nowhere else she wants or needs to be. Her place is here, in this mosque, burying her son. Still, my awareness is heightened. Nour doesn't appear to have reached the threshold for an ambulance; she is not critically unwell. She is expressing her grief through panic and pain. She knew that this day would be tough, and that is why she asked for me to be here. I am here for her and for Nadia as they navigate this darkest of moments.

The azan comes to an end. The women mourners around us gather themselves for prayer, rushed and fussing, their black garments flapping, their hands clasped in agony to their faces. A few latecomers arrive, taking it in turns to wash their feet and hands at the fountain in the corner, for once revealing their lower legs, as the all-female environment allows. They are just in time. The imam begins the service. I am sitting too far from the edge of the balcony to be able to see the men's section and what is happening below. The women around me follow the prayers, their lips moving silently. But, occasionally, an uncontrollable expression of grief escapes. A few of the women are using wheelchairs, and I watch them gracefully pray from their confined positions. When one of them drops her prayer beads to the carpet, someone scoops them up and passes them back.

I know the imam cares about young people as much as I do. I want to believe that he prays for young people, wishes them well and appeals for their safety. I hope he prayed for Amir when he was alive, as he does now at his funeral. As the Salat al-Janazah, the prayer for the dead, continues, I wonder if he is now releasing Amir's soul so that he can be with the angels, free from school bullies, free from the tormentors in his neighbourhood.

'From Allah we come, to Allah we return,' the imam intones. 'May Allah forgive him.'

An older woman approaches our gathering, telling us that the mother has been granted permission to view the body before the burial. The time has come. The women and girls around me weep louder, holding their hands out to Allah. For a moment, they seem frozen, a tableau of grief.

As Nour attempts to get to her feet, her knees give way. I support her and she tries again to stand, but again her legs buckle. Facing her, I manage to get my arm underneath hers and, with effort, she rises unsteadily. I am looking at a face that's worn out with grief. I ask her if she wants me to support her during the viewing of the body, and she nods.

The little room where Amir's body is being prepared for burial feels like an endless walk from the women's quarter as we shuffle slowly along. Nour struggles to put one foot in front of the other, even with Nadia holding her hand on her other side to give her strength. We awkwardly inch forward, and this is the first time I have seen Nadia crumble. Tears roll from her eyes and her hands are not free to wipe them away. She is staggering a little. Her cousins and friends are by her side, a wall of grieving women, all supporting each other. I turn to console Nour, but tears are falling down my own cheeks and I have no words.

Amir's body is lying on a raised table; a few men, who must be close family members, are attending to it, washing him with soap and water. My first encounter with a dead body was in my student nursing days, when a ward sister asked me to clean a patient who had died just a few hours earlier. I remember taking my time to put on an apron and gloves; I was so frightened, I wanted to delay the task for as long as possible. Over the years, that fear retreated; instead, I came to recognize the enormous honour of caring for the dead and I stopped being scared. Nursing has prepared me well for this moment, and yet still it's almost unbearable. It is hard to believe that the young boy I used to see in the streets and at the PRU is no longer with us. Death is never soft or easy, but the death of a young person is incomprehensible. It leaves so many questions unanswered.

In the small viewing room, women are slowly filling up the space, squeezing in together so that we can all spend a last moment with Amir. Time slows down; the air is heavy and smells of death. I help Nour move close to her son's body. She seems completely unaware of everyone else in the room. For her, this is an intimate moment with her boy and everyone and everything else recedes. She whispers to him, endless whispers. She kisses him on his forehead, her cracked lips resting gently on his brow. I hope that this is the beginning of her journey to closure, a moment of ease and peace as she releases her son's spirit. Unresolved grief can lead to dark waters – Nour needs to lean into her grief and make sense of it, otherwise her diabetes and hypertension will further compromise her physical and mental health.

The room is silent, save for the sound of weeping. Then, the men signal that it is enough, that they need to move the body on. It's time to say goodbye to Amir.

'Habibi Amir,' the women whisper to their dear child.

'Allahu akbar,' they whisper.

I take a few deep breaths and look at Amir for the last time. His mouth and eyes are closed, his light brown skin is now ash grey, his cold body has surrendered itself to the afterlife. His long, slim shape is wrapped in a white cloth, a shroud. His head is shaved. I lean over to say something to him.

In my last conversation with Amir, I had allowed silence for mindfulness, encouraging him to reflect on his behaviours, encouraging him to modify them and his responses and reactions to events. Stephen and I had talked to Amir repeatedly about the dangers of getting into fights. He had often shrugged at us, saying that we worried too much. It was a line we heard often from the young people we were working with; their age and vulnerability meant that their judgement of risk and danger was impaired.

They are only children, after all.

'Nurse. I am alright, man. I am alright. I can take care of myself. Go worry about my mum. She's the one who needs you, not me,' he'd said. It was what he always said.

Now, in our final conversation, I thank him for making me the nurse that I am today. Young people like Amir have taught me the art of nursing, the importance of connecting with young people at a human level. They have taught me that violence is not without vulnerability; that the streets may dictate the way young people behave, but their faith is just as powerful an influence; that they love their families and love life. I thank Amir for the opportunity to learn from him, as well as to nurse him.

The women help to get Nour out of the room. I try to hold onto her arm, but I lose my grip. I feel someone gently moving me on, nudging me out of this space and out of the mosque. As we exit, a roiling mass of bodies, Nour and Nadia are swept into a waiting car. I watch as it moves slowly away, Nadia's tall headwrap clearly visible through the back window. They are heading to the burial site, where my attendance is not appropriate. I linger around the exit as other mourners start to gather around the hearse that will be carrying Amir's body. Young people take pictures and videos on their phones – not to humiliate Amir this time, but to honour his spirit and the joy he brought to this world in his short life. I look up at the sky as a flock of birds – starlings, I think – fly in formation over the mosque, as if in send-off. As the hearse departs, the mosque clears as quickly as it had filled up, the crowd scattering every which way. Unnoticed, I make my way out onto the street.

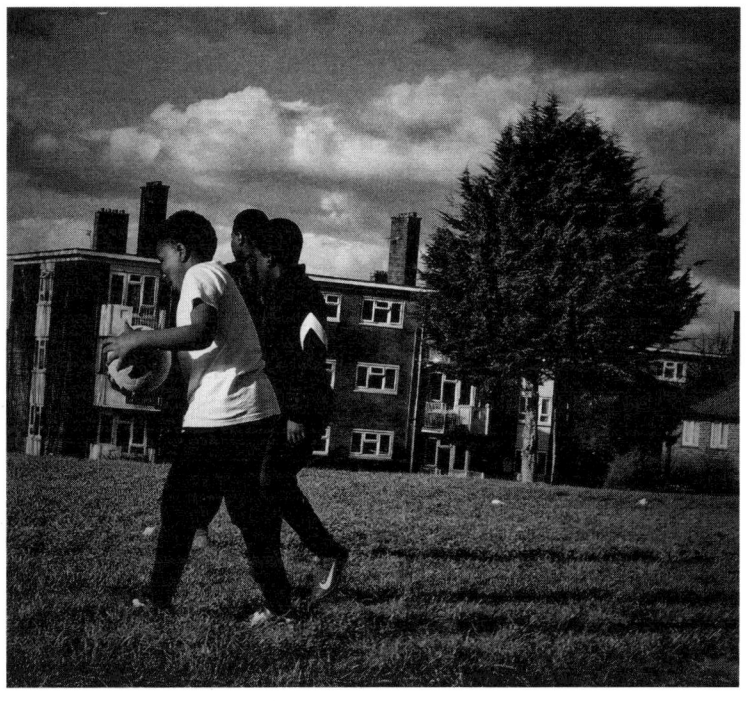

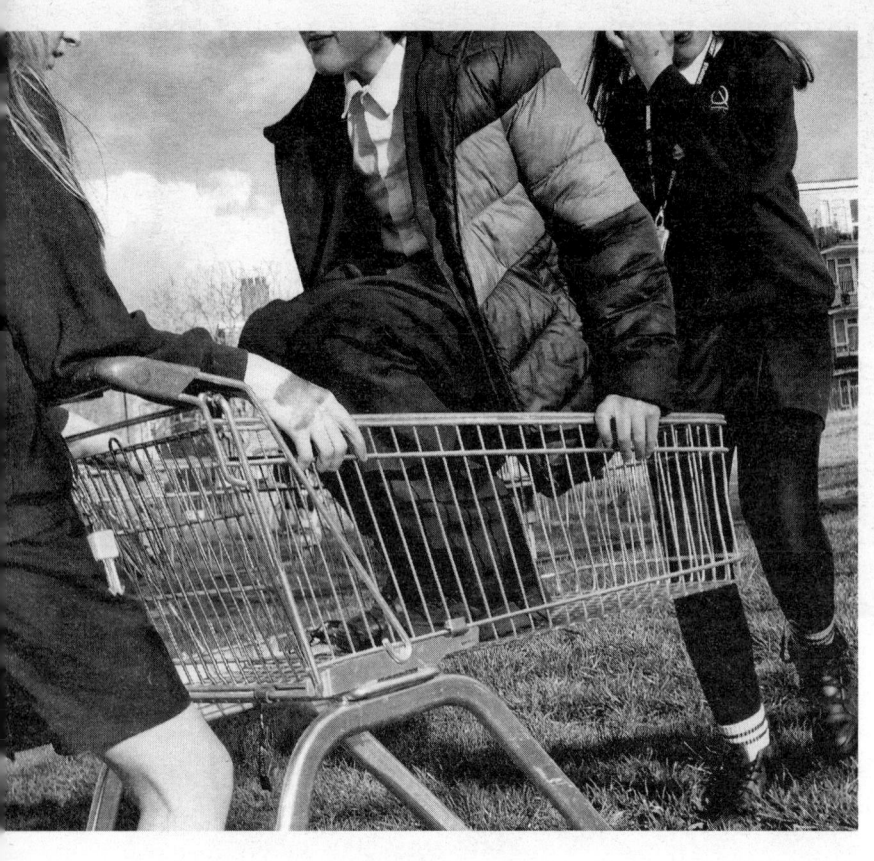

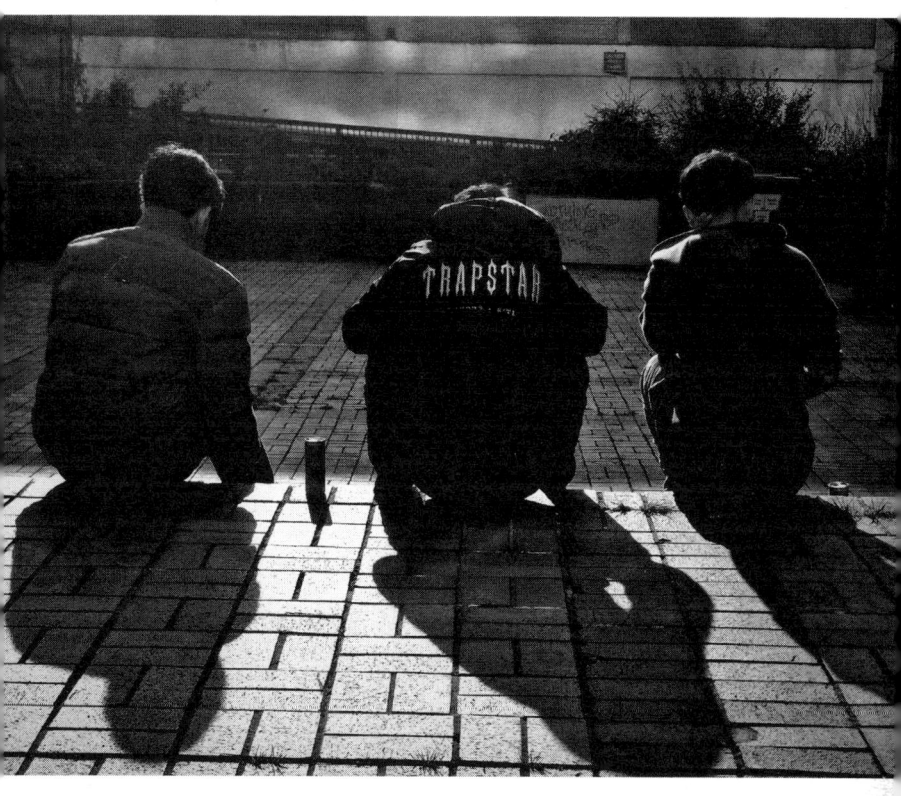

The sun is beginning to set, and I no longer feel safe walking along the canal, which, at night, is riddled with petty crime and drug dealing. Instead, I head south on the main road, bending to tie my laces next to a closed iron gate that leads to private parkland. It has always bothered me that so much of London's open space is closed off to the public, excluding the very people that most need access to it. Where on earth are teenagers like Amir supposed to play, if so much of London is inaccessible to them?

As I walk, I think about Nour and Nadia and their new reality beyond the funeral and the crowds, the well-wishers and the solidarity they're experiencing today. What will it be like when they return to their flat and find themselves hemmed in on all sides by the same issues that swallowed Amir and took him to his grave? Nadia has often talked about her dreams of leaving the estate. She is bright and understands that she lives in one of London's wealthiest boroughs and yet, in her own estate, people are struggling to keep their heads above water. She's told me she wonders if Amir would have survived if they had lived in a different part of London, or perhaps a community on the outskirts, a suburb where life feels safer. She will never know.

What Nadia does know is that she doesn't want to be defined by her brother's activities. They are not the same person. Yet his actions have become the family's signature; they have become known as a 'troubled family', people to be avoided. Nadia has told me that she pursued law because she wants to understand how the law works against young people – rather than for them – particularly those from working-class backgrounds, whose heritage lies beyond the UK. She wants to try to change things and make life better for people like her. People like Amir.

I have to hope that, now the worst thing that can happen has happened, she will have the strength to succeed.

5. Jordan: The Church

'When gang members embrace religion, it creates a conflict that forces individuals to choose either gang or religious life. Choosing religion is a step toward gang disengagement and reductions in criminal behaviour.'

THE GOOD FRIDAY SERVICE at the Pentecostal church in south London's Elephant and Castle is in full swing when I arrive. I could hear the excitable beat of drums and the sound of soulful voices long before I found the discreet front door of the community hall. A middle-aged man and a younger woman are standing just inside the doorway, and are polite and welcoming. The man speaks softly, with a faint African accent I can't quite place, and asks if I am new to church. But before I can find the right words to answer him – to say that I am new to *this* church, but not to *the* Church – the woman ushers me inside to join the unexpectedly large congregation. There is no time for small talk – and, anyway, the greeters' words would be swallowed up by the swell of voices. The woman's hurried movements as she gestures for me to take a seat suggest that I will not want to miss a moment more. Before returning to the door, she hands me a small glossy leaflet; I look down to see a modern illustration of a Black Christ tied to a cross, his head hanging loosely, his blood represented by digital red lines. The caption reads: *For us he gave his life.*

The choir, dressed in white and green, is positioned at the front of the congregation, the rapt faces of the worshippers looking on. Men, women, young adults – all of life is represented here. Even as the sound of the music subsides, it's a performance I can't tear my eyes from. The pastor – Pastor Obi, I will later gather – is in early middle-age, and he stands in the midst of the choir on a long, raised platform; he is wearing a microphone headset like a rock star presiding over a festival crowd. As he begins to speak over the choir's now subdued backing, he paces up and down the podium, his chest rising and falling with every emphatic word. The congregation is alive, festive, fizzing with energy, their colourful outfits lighting up the drab hall. Women in beautiful figure-hugging dresses swing their hips in sensual rhythm. Attuned to the pastor's sermon now, a number of people are humming and whispering, responding to each word. I hear mumblings of 'Yes, Jesus' and 'To the blood of Christ'. A few people begin speaking in tongues. As the choir's singing becomes strong again, and their bodies move with increasing rhythm, their collective voice brings the dreary space to life. A few of the congregation approach the podium to be nearer to their pastor. Many have their arms in the air, palms raised in spiritual surrender.

I am here to meet Auntie Florence, seventeen-year-old Jordan's grandmother, a defiant and dignified Malawian woman who has been his guardian since his birth, and is the closest thing he has to a mother figure. We have been trying to meet for some time, and securing a meeting with her has been difficult, but it is important; her grandson has been referred, through the Gangs Unit, to my clinic for mental-health and trauma care. He has been involved in petty crime for a while and is slowly moving up the ranks of gang activity. Since he was stabbed a few months ago, he has become even more volatile and aggressive.

Rather than scaring him, the episode has brought out the fighter in him, but that Jordan is both a victim and a perpetrator of violence is clear to me. His key worker, Miles, has given me a briefing on the complexity of the case and feels that I can also add some value to the mental-health needs of Jordan's family.

Many professionals have tried to work with Auntie Florence over the past few months and it has been difficult for all of them. She has become well known for rejecting white social workers out of hand. Race and spirituality are important issues for her. She argues that, without these qualities, how could anyone possibly understand her world? She has very clear values, and very clear boundaries around who she chooses to associate with. Sometimes those values are compatible with the system, but often they are not. Too often, we place the blame for these relationship breakdowns on the client; we complain that they're being difficult, that they are 'hard to reach'. The failure to connect means that the core issues of vulnerability and mental health are never addressed and the problems persist, but the failure is ours too.

I have been asked to work on the case in the hope that I can make a difference to Jordan's downward trajectory; my ethnicity and my faith matter a great deal to Auntie Florence.

Pinning Jordan down to a meeting has been equally difficult; he has perfected a way of declining invitations ever so politely, gently insisting that he doesn't need any help. Not for the first time, the young person I'm here for has told me that, rather than helping *them*, it's their loved one who needs my support, the stress of their child's behaviour having become too great for them. Jordan has proved himself to be particularly strategic; he doesn't mind me coming to his home, but is always quick to divert my attention away from himself and towards his grandmother. Auntie Florence has problems with her blood pressure; sometimes she takes her tablets, but sometimes she doesn't.

She's not sleeping well. She's losing weight. At our last meeting, I suggested to Jordan that perhaps we could both help to keep Auntie Florence's blood pressure down by working together to address how some of his behaviours are affecting her health. But he continues to push back. No progress is being made. If my nursing interventions are going to have any impact on Jordan, it's clear that I need to strike up a strong and trusting relationship with Auntie Florence.

'Which country are you from?' she asked me abruptly the first time we met in their small flat, surrounded by her children and other grandchildren. Then: 'Which church do you go to?'

I rumbled on about growing up in a colonial Rhodesia, now Zimbabwe, and attending a Methodist church there, the branch of Christianity founded by John Wesley, the British colonial theorist who spread his theological teachings throughout southern Africa in the eighteenth century. Today, people who attend the Methodist church are known locally as 'Mawhisiri', a word that rhymes with Wesley's name. As I talked with Auntie Florence, I remembered the many charitable moments of the services of my childhood, when a giving bowl would be passed around the congregation as the choir sang. People would contribute what they could, if they could. No one was under any obligation. Mawhisiri, I said to Auntie Florence, are renowned for their joyful singing, generous charity and concise church services.

Satisfied with my answers, we performed the little dance of getting to know each other. Auntie Florence asked me how long I'd been a nurse. She wanted to know if I worked for the NHS or for social services, a distinction that's important to her. She was wary of social services, she told me. Many of my families are. We talked a little about Jordan, who had already slipped out of the room. But she seemed reluctant to share too much in case the rest of the family was listening in – in such a small space it was impossible for them not to. I got the impression she wanted to protect Jordan and I respected that.

'If you want to see me, come to church,' she repeatedly said. 'Come at Easter, on Good Friday. We will be praising the Lord.'

It wasn't an invitation. It was an instruction.

*

I got to know Elephant and Castle well when I lived in Brixton, many years ago. Certain pockets of south London have always been rich in African and Caribbean culture, beginning with the Windrush generation, who began to settle here in the late 1940s, followed by West African and, more recently, South American communities. In the years that I lived in south London, Brixton was shunned by those who weren't local or didn't understand it. But the area holds so much history. It's a vibrant, creative hub. Renowned artists have played gigs there and have been influenced by its Caribbean culture. The graffiti which decorates the busy streets is a celebration of a community that has borne witness to some of the best and worst of London, from the Brixton riots of 1981, sparked by conflicts between the police and the locals, to the passing of the London Olympic torch in 2012. The Black community in Brixton and south London as a whole is made up of defiant, resilient and colourful people, and there is never a dull moment when one is among them.

And so, here I am, at the Pentecostal church, looking for Auntie Florence, running a little late, but immediately caught up in a joyful atmosphere of worship that excites me. The congregation exudes a sense of freedom. There are tears of joy, and a feeling of healing and spiritual identity. This is the space in which Jordan has grown up, and which Auntie Florence still hopes will heal him. A space where community values, morality, hope, self-esteem and self-improvement are preached at full throttle. Auntie Florence loves her church and believes in its

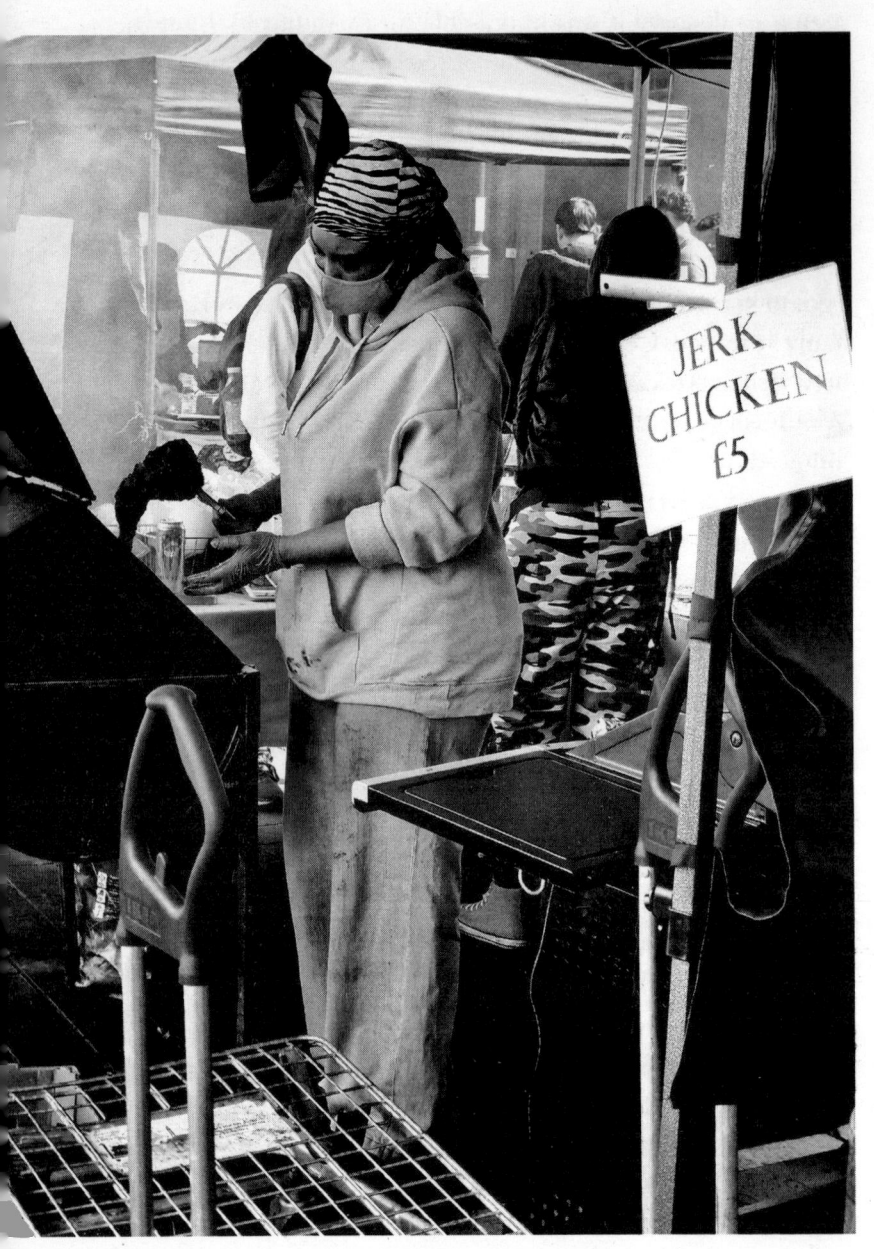

power to do good. And yet it is having absolutely no influence over Jordan's worrying trajectory. How has he has ended up on the streets, so far removed from all that is safe or spiritual?

I begin to move through the congregation, apologizing and excusing myself, all the while looking for Auntie Florence. It doesn't take long to spot her. Today, her house dress and apron are nowhere to be seen. She is wearing an elegant green chitenge, a glamorous fabric predominantly worn by women in southern and eastern Africa, similar to a sarong. Her bold earrings are a nod to Malawi, her country of origin. Her shimmering top, a light shade of brown, hugs at the waist. Her hands have risen into the air, as if involuntarily; she seems to be in a trance, immersed in fervent prayer.

As the choir's song recedes again, Pastor Obi asks if anyone is facing any challenges in their lives that they would like the congregation to pray for. He encourages people to come to him and they begin to gather in the central aisle. As people arrange themselves, Pastor Obi moves the focus of the prayer on to more global issues. He prays for those in the Democratic Republic of Congo who have not known peace for too many years now, for children living with disease and hunger around the world, for peace in the Middle East. Then he turns his focus to local issues. He prays for the Black community to find peace with ourselves, to avoid those things that seek to divide us.

He is a powerful orator, and his ability to persuade, plead with and influence the congregation is evident in the honour they give him. I'm distracted by the thought that the entire body of religion is plagued by controversy and ethical dilemmas, but, as I listen to him and watch how his words are landing with his devout congregation, I can't help but hope that the pastor is preaching within the boundaries of what he can actually influence. That he isn't overpromising.

As if feeding off my anxieties, Pastor Obi goes on. He will

pray for those with marital problems so that those marriages can thrive again. He will heal anyone with drug and alcohol problems and enable them to walk away from the toxic evils that prey on their minds and bodies. He will heal those with fertility problems so that they will bear children – lots of children. He will heal those with disabilities. He prays for the children and young people who are worried about knife crime, and for those who have died because of it. He has observed the suffering within the community, he tells us, and prays that the suffering might end. Finally, his prayers embrace those without money, and he tells them that, if they pray hard enough, Jesus will bless them with money, and he draws on examples of people who have miraculously gained wealth in this manner.

I have faith, but I am also sceptical. How on earth can the pastor pray for people who are facing such enormous problems and dare to offer them false hope? It strikes me that Auntie Florence, frozen in rapture, may well be praying for Jordan, and is probably hoping that, by some process of osmosis, the pastor's words will reach Jordan and influence his behaviour. But prayer alone can't fix these problems. Jordan is going to need much more than prayers to help with the predicament he has found himself in.

I find myself shaking my head.

An older man unsteady on his feet has joined the group in the aisle, and leans heavily on his walking stick. It seems those before the altar all believe their problems are about to be solved. They are deep in prayer, some holding pictures of their loved ones, some with young children in their arms who look bewildered by the goings-on. Many are women – women of all ages – and this speaks to something, I realize. Are there so many of them because they carry the heaviest burden of society's challenges? Does that sense of responsibility make them more likely to seek help in this spiritual space? And does their desperate need make them more vulnerable to exploitation by the very institution they have turned to in their hour of need?

A contribution pot is in circulation and members of the congregation are offering up their donations. There are a lot of people here; it seems to me like a lot of money. I watch from a distance as Auntie Florence pushes a fold of twenty-pound notes into the large receptable. I estimate it's a contribution of maybe a hundred pounds.

Auntie Florence works as a cleaner in a hotel in central London. She lives in council accommodation. How is she able to afford this? Churches with African and Caribbean roots are thriving, while white congregations are dwindling. Black churches are a success story in what is otherwise an increasingly secular society. I'm worried that the church is exploiting Auntie Florence's vulnerability, and that of so many others like her – people whose lives are challenging and difficult, who find it impossible to put their trust in the police or the schools or the NHS, and instead turn passionately to God. But, if this is where people find solace, who am I to question it?

Church has great symbolic meaning in Black culture the world over. For London's African communities, it is a place of sanctuary, of community, fellowship, worship and love. Strangers who become friends who become family meet here, under the common umbrella of a revered God. At their best, churches offer much more than the salvation of the soul. They're socio-religious spaces that provide people with safety, shelter and hope by addressing the pertinent issues affecting communities. It's not surprising that the pastor has included the issue of knife crime in his list of afflictions. He's well aware of the impact deaths from stabbings have on his congregation. And it's precisely the reason why Auntie Florence might be finding comfort within this particular church – and is happy to pay for it.

I move closer to the front of the church in the hope of

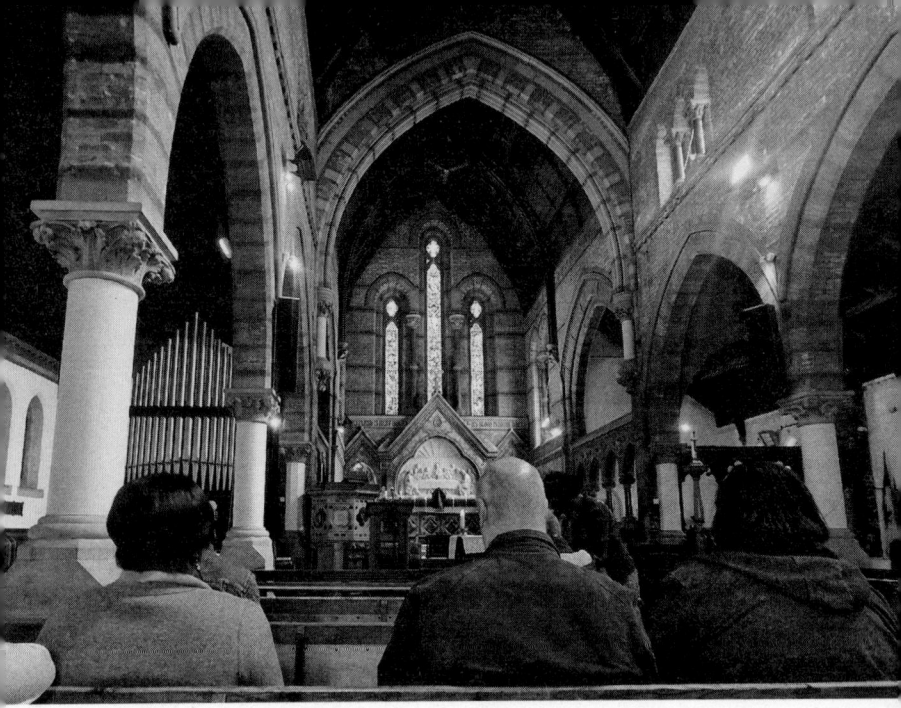

catching Auntie Florence's eye; as she emerges from her reverie, I get lucky. She gazes in my direction and her glazed eyes find focus. But, instead of peace, I see worry there. She is on the verge of tears. She seems troubled.

*

Later in the service, I find a seat beside Auntie Florence, and she turns to me.

'How are you?' she whispers, tapping the back of my hand.

'I am fine, thank you,' I say, although I am not entirely confident of that. Something about the lack of emotional control in the hall concerns me. The ecstasy, the moaning and the speaking in tongues are beyond the scope of my nursing skills. I am out of my comfort zone. 'How are *you*, Auntie Florence?' I ask in return. 'How is Jordan?'

'Jordan is at home. I have prayed for him. The pastor has prayed for him too,' she tells me, with an assurance that suggests those heartfelt prayers will settle all concerns for Jordan's questionable well-being and his uncertain future. 'The church can help me to heal Jordan,' she goes on. 'All I need to do is bring him here for one service and pay some money to the pastor.'

I blink, searching for words. But for a moment we are both distracted by the choir, whose voices soar once again. The pastor is preaching in tongues, as if in personal conversation with God; the space between heaven and earth just became narrower, as if one could pass through and be safely delivered.

I frown and Auntie Florence moves closer to me, as if to comfort my worrying mind. She touches my arm. The warmth of her motherly hand feels good.

'The pastor has said that Jordan can be delivered from the problems he is having,' she whispers to me. She looks more confident now, but I am much less certain.

'*How* will Jordan be delivered from his problems?' I ask. 'Did the pastor say how?'

The service has reached an end, and people are gathering their possessions, rising from their seats and beginning to move towards the exit. Auntie Florence begins to stand too.

I don't move, still waiting for her answer. But no answer comes. Instead, she holds my hand and, with a squeeze, says, 'Come and meet Pastor Obi.'

She stops to say hello to a few people along the way, each greeting evolving into a short conversation enquiring into the well-being of various family members. All the while, Auntie Florence holds onto my hand. I am transported back to Zimbabwe. I am a little girl once again, holding onto my mother's frock while she moves gracefully around the church, fully at ease, catching up with her many friends.

But something about this whole experience is making me

feel deeply uncomfortable. I'm unable to separate some of my own residual issues with the Church from the feeling of goodwill that floods this space, and I am aware that this could be getting in the way of achieving the goal before me. This incredible institution, which offers some so much spiritual hope, also leaves room for so much manipulation, exploitation and abuse. The poor are most susceptible, and too many churches will take their money even when they know there is nothing left for them to give. I am concerned that Auntie Florence can't afford to give money to the church, that it will drive her further into poverty. She can't afford to put all her faith in Pastor Obi. He alone cannot deliver Jordan from evil. For the moment, however, I put my fears and frustrations to one side and meekly follow in Auntie Florence's tiny footsteps.

We eventually find ourselves at the back of the hall, and I can see Pastor Obi standing to the side of a table laid out with Bibles for purchase. There's a queue building; people are waiting to speak to him. The small crowd is patient, orderly, whispering among themselves to pass the time, but their eyes are watching the pastor's every movement, waiting for their turn. When Auntie Florence and I are eventually awarded a moment with him, and he hears that I am a mental-health nurse, he gets straight into the issues.

'You know, we have problems with these young people everywhere. In Brixton, Stockwell, Clapham, Croydon. The problem is everywhere,' he says.

Auntie Florence nods along, hanging on his every word.

'We lost one of our young people last year,' he continues. 'A twenty-year-old boy, shot dead in Peckham. A month after that, another boy was stabbed in Camberwell.'

The pastor moves his Bible into his right hand and, with his left, takes my elbow and pulls me closer to him, his voice quieter now.

'Nurse, two years ago, we buried my nephew. Seventeen years old, bright boy, an A student. He could have gone to Oxford, Cambridge, anything at all that he wanted. But he was stabbed to death, by his own friend. His mother has never recovered. She can never recover. That made me want to do something about it.' His voice is low and trembling, a startling contrast to the preacher who stood before us moments ago, but his hand on my arm feels forceful.

I lean away, his grip easing off as I put distance between us, and gently ask what it is he's doing.

He tells me that he went to a prayer conference in the US where they talked about healing for communities affected by violence, that he is now able to help his own community through prayer and fasting, and that he can do this for a small fee.

'How much do people have to pay?' I ask the pastor.

'It's not much, my dear, not much at all,' Auntie Florence slips into the conversation. 'Pastor Obi is helping us. He is helping me with Jordan's situation.'

I am moved by Pastor Obi's story, and by his commitment to his congregation. And yet I can't help but wonder what he does with the money they contribute.

'Can you help without making the congregation pay?' I ask Pastor Obi.

I can feel Auntie Florence glaring at me and I dare not look her way.

I have visions of pastors around the globe who live in mansions and drive around in expensive cars, able to hire or even own helicopters, unashamedly flaunting their obscene wealth even as their congregations are submerged in poverty and misery.

'The money is a calling from God,' Pastor Obi tells me in a level voice. 'It's not so much,' he adds confidently.

I am flabbergasted. I want to know his success rate. I want to know how many families have actually been helped as a result of prayer. I have many questions, but my tongue is tied.

'But most of the people who are struggling with these problems don't have much money,' I finally stutter.

'Now, Nurse Dorcas, you can't say things like that to the pastor,' Auntie Florence hisses at me, squeezing my hand. She looks into my eyes – the same look an African parent gives a child when they are in trouble. I know I have overstepped the mark. I can't compromise my relationship with Auntie Florence, so I step back.

'Auntie Florence, thank you for your contribution today. We will pray for your grandson in Jesus' name,' Pastor Obi says as he moves to the next congregant.

I have been dismissed.

As Auntie Florence says her final farewells, it dawns on me that keeping Jordan and his grandmother safe has just become exponentially harder. I do not trust Pastor Obi. This level of exploitation will take time to unpick. But I am committed to the work, however difficult.

*

Like many other organizations, the multi-agency team that I work with recognizes the complexity of the work that we do and its impact on our own well-being. I check into our regular systemic therapy session, which is run by Clinton, a highly able and experienced psychotherapist with a background in youth violence and psychology. I discuss Jordan's case with my colleagues there, who take much joy from describing their own experiences with their faith, and we talk about the value of collective worship.

'Don't overlook the church. Many good things happen in those churches,' they say to me, almost as one.

They interrogate my approach to Jordan's case, suggesting that perhaps I shouldn't view the church and its activities only through the lens of vulnerability and exploitation, but should remember that it provides a strong community cohesion. It is a place of psychological safety for many in its congregation and it's that robust unity which I should be harnessing to shape my interventions with Jordan and Auntie Florence. They encourage me to recognize the good work that the church is doing to address youth violence and knife crime in the community and suggest that there is scope for us as a team to offer Black-majority churches, like Auntie Florence's, workshops on mental health and knife crime, so that people have the facts at their fingertips, not just a prayer offered up to their God.

The group then questions my personal views about the Church to see whether my own experience may be getting in the way. They have a point. When a colleague asks me why I felt so triggered by the visit, I have to pause to gather my thoughts. It's the first time in a while that I have felt vulnerable with my team members, but I also feel safe enough to go with it. I find my voice and start to talk about my early experiences as an immigrant from Zimbabwe living in south London, where I attended a Pentecostal church at the suggestion of a friend. I was welcomed into the congregation and was then very quickly encouraged to give 10 per cent of my salary as a tithe. At the time, I was working as a healthcare assistant in a mental-health hospital in central London, earning just enough to meet my basic needs. Understandably, I was reluctant to pay the money. I began to reduce my attendance and eventually stopped going entirely. A few of the church leaders hounded me to come back, but my view was that the church wasn't meeting my spiritual needs. Rather, they seemed entirely focused on taking a share of my earnings. My presence there wasn't about me, it was about them.

Being in church with Auntie Florence had brought back some of these conflicted emotions: a sense of duty to God, hard up against a greater sense of doubt about the people acting as His representatives.

My colleagues validate my feelings, but also offer caution; I shouldn't allow my personal experience of the Church to overshadow the important work of addressing the mental-health needs of Jordan and Auntie Florence, which, if executed well, could help to steer Jordan away from gang activity and keep him safe.

Armed with a far greater clarity, I leave the meeting feeling much better equipped to proceed with the case. Energized, and full of all sorts of creative ideas about how to go forward, I'm itching to get on with it.

*

A month after my Pentecostal church attendance, I'm back in south London, emerging out of Brixton Tube station to clouds pregnant with early summer rains. I'm meeting Jordan in Coldharbour Lane for coffee, his preferred place to see me. We have been texting each other for weeks now, trying to arrange a date. He has been evasive, but I have finally been able to pin him down.

On my journey, I have been listening to a podcast about how climate change is affecting urban cities and spaces, which has got me thinking about how recent government policies have steadily reduced public meeting places previously accessible to young people like Jordan, who are among those impacted by these cutbacks. Something needs to be done to rectify this, because where else is there for them to congregate other than on the streets?

The Caribbean man who has been standing outside the Tube station every day for years now, preaching the Bible, is in place. No one seems to mind. No one seems to care. I note once again the vibrant colours and bustle of the market. I notice, too, how

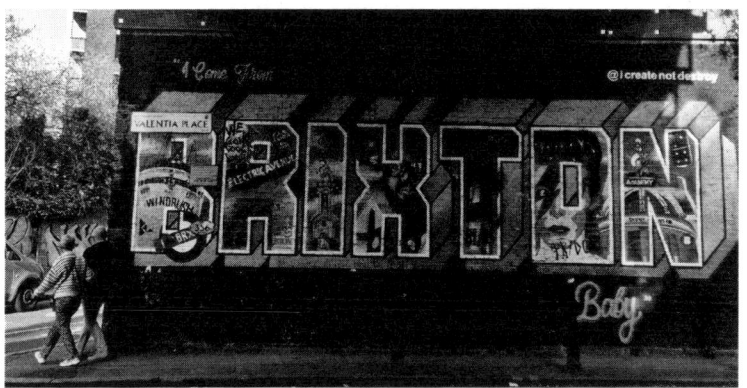

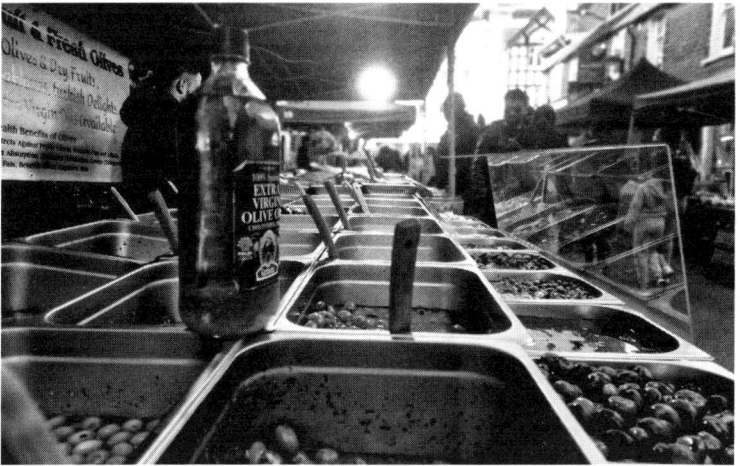

the demographics in Brixton have changed since I lived here. In recent years, regeneration and gentrification have ushered in a whiter, more middle-class community, and the property prices have been pushed up. Some of the area's multiculturalism has been muted. The locals who remain vent about how a cup of coffee used to cost two pounds but now costs five. They are being priced out of the area. The result is a sort of segregation that can be isolating and excluding for those Black people who remain; there's a growing sense of 'them' and 'us'. I'm grateful for people like Auntie Florence, for whom Brixton will always be home.

I grab a seat at an Ethiopian cafe nestled on a side street and dutifully fork out. When Jordan emerges from the crowds, he looks remarkably relaxed, and I see he's wearing a uniform of sorts: a black T-shirt onto which the rap artist Tupac's face is printed. I notice he has a few other young boys in tow. At a push, they might be fifteen, sixteen. Less relaxed, they wear their hoods up and they're anxiously looking around. Body language alone tells me that they look up to Jordan – he is their leader. There's reverence in their demeanour. This, I realize, is also a kind of worship and fellowship; the layers of power and vulnerability are clear.

Jordan can tell that I'm confused, that my mind is busy trying to understand the dynamics of the group.

'These are my boys, innit, Auntie Dorcas,' he says as he reaches me, the young men forming a scrappy circle around him. His voice is harsh, edgy, authoritative. It's a stark contrast to the respectful behaviour I know he's capable of and which he exhibits when he's home, among his family.

In response, I nod curtly. I am not impressed.

Jordan gives a signal to his boys and they move away from us, but not too far. Not far enough. I can see them hovering just around the corner.

'How are you, Jordan?' I say, finally getting to check in with him.

His eyes look tired, but he's alert and doesn't appear to be under the influence of drugs or alcohol. But something is clearly bothering him.

'I am alright, you know, Auntie.' He gestures over his shoulder to his friends. 'Since I got stabbed, I move around with these guys, innit.'

'How are these boys helping you since you got stabbed, Jordan?' I ask pointedly.

'They look out for me, innit.'

My mind is doing summersaults. Jordan's keyworker, Miles, hasn't briefed me about Jordan's changing friendships or the new measures he has adopted to keep himself safe since the stabbing. Jordan appears to have recruited some followers to add a layer of protection. What that means in reality is that he may well be exploiting these young boys to his benefit. It feels oddly similar to the situation with Pastor Obi, who I feel is exploiting Auntie Florence and indeed the rest of his congregation. This situation seems similarly out of my control.

I need to take the time to understand Jordan. Who *is* he?

Jordan, I see, plays the streets very differently from the way he plays his home environment. At home, he is a child. But the streets are his territory, where he expects to have control. He has eyes and ears on the streets; his brethren take the temperature and give warning of danger. Like a pack of hunting dogs, they have power and presence in their numbers. At home, he is just his nan's boy, her beloved grandson. In her eyes, he can do no wrong – any harm that has come to him has been because of other people, not his own actions. Auntie Florence sees only innocence in him – Jordan as the victim – so much so that she believes any bad behaviours are negligible issues that can be forgiven by the church. But Jordan is no longer the kind of person who goes to church. The streets are his church now, and reconciling this reality with Auntie Florence's expectations will be a challenge.

I think about the situation in terms of nursing interventions; I can only work with what is within my nursing scope. I am keen to explore how the stabbing is impacting on Jordan's mental well-being and to get some sense of how he is using the young ones to manage his anxieties about the streets. This will be useful information for Miles. But, before I can begin, Jordan once again takes charge of the conversation. He is strategic and purposeful. It dawns on me that I am being played.

'Tell Nan that I would love to come to church, but I can't, innit,' he says to me, as though I too am one of his boys, here to do his bidding.

The reason he can't come to church, even if he wanted to, he tells me, is because he can't cross postcode lines into Elephant and Castle. That's where he got stabbed.

'Nan is at her wits' end worrying about you,' I say to him. 'She is praying for you.'

Jordan nods. He is aware that prayers are being said for him. 'Tell Nan that, out here, it don't work like that. You don't go to church to sort out your problems. You sort them out here, on the street, innit.' He emphasizes the point by gesturing to the pavement: 'here' is the ground beneath our feet, a postcode, a borough.

'What exactly is it that you feel you need to sort out on the streets, Jordan?' I ask.

His silence speaks to the fear and uncertainty he's feeling. I know that Jordan is scared for his life; the need to protect himself weighs heavily on his seventeen-year-old shoulders. I am his mental-health nurse; I'm here to lessen the traumatic burden, but I am struggling to burrow my way into the depth of his emotions.

I acknowledge his request for me to pass on a message to his nan, but I also suggest that he have a word with her himself. I can see that he's reluctant to do that. Perhaps he doesn't want to hurt her feelings. Or maybe, aged just seventeen, he's simply not able to navigate his grandmother's obsession with the church. And I can at least understand that.

'What do you most fear, Jordan?' I ask him, my voice lowered, leaning across the cups of coffee between us.

It's a question that clearly hits hard. His shoulders drop and his posture immediately becomes less imposing. I have taken a chip out of his ego. The child returns. We sit in silence, save for the market traders touting for business. Brixton seems to stand still.

'I fear a lot, Auntie Dorcas. I fear death. I fear God . . . I fear everything,' he eventually says. 'But I can't show it, innit.'

I know that he has only been able to say this because he feels a sense of safety and trust between us. Jordan is reaching out for help.

'Lot of people getting stabbed. Some are dead, just like that,' he mutters with a flick of his fingers and a shake of his head. 'I worry about that.'

Jordan shares that, since he was stabbed, he has been having flashbacks to the incident. The whole episode is made more traumatic by the fact that the person who stabbed him was a friend of his, someone he trusted. Since the stabbing, he hasn't been sleeping well. He finds it difficult to put his faith in others and his recruiting of the 'youngers' is his way of trying to feel in control in a situation that he has no control over.

With a wave of the hand, Jordan signals to the youngers that he needs more time with me, that he will catch up with them later. They disappear into the Brixton crowds. I am relieved that they are gone, albeit into an unsafe world.

'Are you not worried about one of your youngers getting stabbed in your name?' I ask Jordan. I am operating on the edge, here, entering into territory that is way beyond my remit. But it's important to discuss how Jordan's personal risks are pulling the most vulnerable into danger too.

'Yeah, I think about it, Auntie. Course I do,' he says, not meeting my eyes.

I wonder if he feels the weight of responsibility that he should as the guardian of these young boys, and how the youngers' parents feel about their children taking off with Jordan. I want to probe deeper on the issues of power and exploitation, but this is not my area. I have to leave it to Miles. I have to keep within the scope of my mental-health work, to that which is measurable and achievable. In any case, it's a line of questioning that has made Jordan uncomfortable, and I feel he'll want to leave if I pursue it further.

Bringing the focus back to his mental health, we work out some action points together. I agree to continue supporting Auntie Florence. Jordan agrees to talk to Miles about his youngers, and how his fears about his safety might better be mitigated. He also agrees to meet me again – we're going to explore his trauma from the stabbing and work out how he can adopt better ways of coping with his anxiety.

Soon, Jordan disappears into the Brixton crowds. While I'm satisfied that progress has been made, I can't help but worry about his safety, about losing him to the streets. I too fear the worst, that he'll get stabbed again, but fatally this time. It's a chilling possibility. And I worry about what that would do to Auntie Florence.

*

I discuss the progress I've made with Miles. He suggests that we offer the church a workshop on knife crime, trauma and healing, in which we can address issues of vulnerability, mental health, early signs of gang involvement and how to protect children. Keeping an open mind, we also agree to work directly with Pastor Obi to address the fears the community has about losing their children to knife crime, creating an open-space dialogue with the congregation, particularly those working with children, and providing an outlet for their grief.

It's an offer that's well received. Auntie Florence and the

pastor feel that a workshop will be a good fit, that it is aligned with some of their biblical teaching around parenting and resolving conflicts. There is a specific request from the pastor that we address the issue of culture in the workshop; he feels it's important for families to be allocated professionals who understand their backgrounds. I wonder if this is where Auntie Florence's very vocal preference for Black social workers has come from.

A Saturday morning when most of the congregation will be able to attend is earmarked for the workshop. Auntie Florence agrees to speak about her experiences with Jordan, experiences which she has previously tried hard not to acknowledge. As our common sense of purpose gathers momentum, I feel more at ease and less anxious about the role of the church. I am starting to feel like part of the community, part of a collective that is genuinely concerned about the safety and well-being of its young people. And it feels good.

*

Over the next couple of weeks, there are various text messages between me and Auntie Florence and Jordan, and that's encouraging, but I am keen to catch up with Auntie Florence in person. Although she has responded positively to the workshop, I am still concerned she might be angry with me for interrogating Pastor Obi's financial intentions. The only way to find out how she really feels is to catch up with her in her natural habitat.

'Come and see me at the market on Saturday, when I do my shopping,' she says to me when she picks up my call. 'Come to the market.'

It's an instruction rather than a request, and we make a firm plan for the weekend. But, the next day, I get a text from her.

Jordan is at the police station, it says. *They pick him up last night. Please come and see him, he is asking for you.*

I pause to think, then reach out to Miles. I need to speak to him before rushing in. Miles has managed many young people in custody and in prisons, some of them serving lengthy sentences. He knows the dynamics, the challenges, but most importantly the opportunities that confined environments create for higher-level engagement with young people.

He already knows more than I do about Jordan's situation, telling me he has been arrested for shoplifting and possession of cannabis. He agrees to meet me outside the custody centre where Jordan is being held. I let Auntie Florence know that Miles and I will be there soon.

The custody suite is situated in an unassuming central-London side street. Besides the clutch of homeless people who always congregate outside, there's nothing much to indicate that this is an operational police building. Auntie Florence is already waiting outside when we arrive, pacing to and fro by the front steps. She is holding a Bible and whispering to herself in prayer. She reaches out and grasps my hand as I approach her. Her grip is tight. She's trembling and short of breath – the hypertension from which she suffers is putting a huge strain on her body.

'He was caught stealing,' she tells me, with difficulty. 'Jordan has no reason to steal; he has everything at home.'

She tells us that she has already been inside the custody suite to see Jordan, that it's as if he's a child again, small and embarrassed, devastated by his own actions. He's feeling enormous guilt for the stress he has caused her. This is not the first time that Auntie Florence has had to come to a custody suite to see Jordan. But, although every time it happens he is torn to pieces by her evident pain, he doesn't seem to be able to walk away from his own destructive behaviours. When Auntie Florence cried in front of him, she tells me, he tried to reassure her that everything would be fine. But, with every new incident, Auntie

Florence is worried that things will never be 'fine'. She is worried about losing her grandson completely.

'Don't worry too much, Auntie,' Miles jumps in. 'Maybe this is an opportunity for him to turn things around.'

Miles knows that Jordan will be frightened, and he might be able to harness that fear to make Jordan realize things have to change, that this is the moment. I have seen Miles turn trajectories around for even the most challenging of young people and am hoping that a combination of mental-health care and youth-engagement skills can make a difference for Jordan. I don't want to consider what might happen if we fail.

Despite its grim appearance, the custody suite successfully fuses a sense of no-nonsense law enforcement and compassion. The young police officer who greets us takes time to understand who we are and how we support young people, but he does so while refusing to relinquish any authority. He is in control here. Leaving Auntie Florence in the waiting room, he leads us to Jordan's cell, his watchful eyes observing every move we make.

I take it all in. For me, the environment is reminiscent of an old mental-health asylum. There is an industrial feel to it, all hard surfaces and high ceilings and barred windows. In the distance, there's the tortuous sound of a woman screaming. She wants out, but I imagine so does everyone who is locked up in here.

The cell that has been allocated to Jordan is small and sparse, but I'm pleased to see a bed with a surprisingly thick mattress. Jordan is sitting on it, his head bent down between his knees, as if he's folding himself into a ball of shame.

He is crying hard, and it's so unlike him it shocks me.

'I can't do this anymore,' he whispers as soon as he sees us. 'I don't want to do this, innit.'

Miles and I move closer to support him.

When we're all a little calmer, Miles talks to Jordan for

some time, assuring him that the amount of cannabis found in his possession might just meet the criteria for personal use. It's the shoplifting that's more of a worry. If he's charged with theft, he'll be put on a community order and referred to the Youth Offending Team, who he'll then need to engage with for some months. That's if he hasn't violated an existing order. This is not within my nursing domain, but I trust Miles to be on top of it and to seek the right legal advice for Jordan. For now, Miles and I are here to be present and available for Jordan, offering emotional and practical support.

He looks up at me. 'I am sorry. Tell Nan I'm sorry. Tell Nan I'll come to church,' he says, before he lowers his head again.

There is an old African saying: 'When the drum beats at its loudest, it is about to burst.' Jordan is broken, his ego and energy deflated. His loud display of machismo is gone. He has witnessed violence and been a victim of violence, and this is one police arrest too many.

Enough, he is saying.

Jordan has told us that, because he has troubles with some young people from Elephant and Castle, he simply cannot cross postcodes. Miles will need to plan a safe route for Jordan to travel to church. While I know Auntie Florence will be delighted, I am baffled by Jordan's decision to go back to the church. He's the kind of young person who will question anything and everything. He is anti-establishment and anti-police, as most of my young people are. He is used to being in control, and the balance of power is not in his favour in church. And, I can't help but wonder, what on earth will he wear?

Auntie Florence comes up with a solution. She and Jordan will attend another church, which is a safer journey for Jordan. She is prepared to give up her community, friends and her beloved pastor for her grandson.

'You are loved,' Auntie Florence is saying to Jordan.

Life offers all sorts of possibilities, even for someone like Jordan. What path he now chooses and what happens next are not yet clearly defined. Exiting the streets requires a lifestyle change and will involve cutting alliances with his so-called friends and his youngers, who will drift off in another direction and ally themselves with someone else. It means getting up early for college and committing to studies, or getting a job and working hard, or taking a volunteering role that will open up opportunities. It will require Jordan to build trust and confidence in himself and in his community.

As I walk with Auntie Florence to the bus stop, I sense that this particular horror story is coming to an end and that there is, for once, hope.

*

A week later I message Jordan to arrange to meet and he immediately suggests that I come to his home to see Auntie Florence too. The dial has shifted.

As I walk from the Tube to their flat, I'm thinking about the power of possibilities, how big things can come from the smallest actions. Nothing is constant; violence, fear and trauma are not static. With the right support, transformation can impact

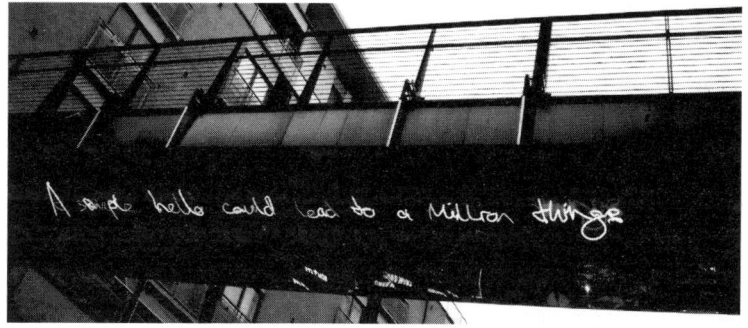

multiple people in one go. The agents of change are not necessarily the big companies pumping money into so-called good causes, performative and disengaged, nor even the politicians of all stripes who make big promises they're unable or unwilling to keep. It's communities themselves which hold the power of change in their hands. If only we could all see that more clearly and use our power more wisely.

'We are cooking!' Auntie Florence says to me as she opens her front door. 'Have you ever had chicken in peanut butter? That's our special dish.'

I shake my head.

'Come and eat, come and eat,' she instructs me, opening up her kitchen and, by extension, I realize, her heart.

A smiling Jordan emerges from his bedroom. He's no longer flustered by my presence in their house and by my sharing information with his grandmother. By welcoming me into his personal space, he's signalling that he has found a new path and is at peace with it. And closure for Jordan means closure for Auntie Florence too.

I notice he's wearing a pair of jeans and a crisp white shirt. He looks uncharacteristically smart and he notes my surprise.

'I'm giving a talk with Miles,' he says by way of explanation. 'I'm talking to some schoolkids about the dangers of knife crime, innit.'

I look into his eyes and say, 'Jordan, I am so proud of you. So, so proud of you.' I can hear my voice quiver. I'm so moved, I fear I might be reduced to tears.

'Eh, look at him now, Dorcas,' Auntie Florence says, cutting through the moment with a joke as she pounds yam in a black pot. 'He should get married and leave me alone. I am done with this one.'

There is a pause, and then we all smile.

6. Jevaun: The Football Pitch

> *'Approximately 20 per cent of people identified as being involved in county lines are children. The average age of children involved in county lines drug dealing is 15.8 years old.'*

It's just gone five o'clock on a dark Thursday afternoon in late November. There's a chill in the air and I clutch instinctively at the collar of my winter coat as I emerge out of the Tube station in east London. Strings of Christmas lights wrap every street lamp and give a fuzzy glow to the winter sky. I'm heading to a Somali and Sudanese community event in Newham, which doesn't start until six thirty. The gathering has been organized by a community that is coming together following several recent stabbings and a number of adolescents and young adults going missing. I'm anticipating that emotions will run high.

With increasing drug consumption in London, the local drug lords have saturated the city's markets and are spilling out into the surrounding home counties, such as Kent, Buckinghamshire and Essex. There, they have penetrated whatever existing drugs-trade structure was already in place and are selling their own supply in lucrative quantities. To reach their new buyers effectively, they are using young people, usually those who are most vulnerable, and sometimes as young as twelve years old. Many of these kids are living with neurodivergent conditions – learning difficulties, ADHD, autism – and all too often they have been excluded from school and are already slipping through the cracks, making it easy to recruit them to run the new drug lines.

Commonly known as 'county lines', the drug dealers use phone lines to control the movement and supply of drugs, usually from cities to small towns, from inner London to the home counties. They do this by exploiting vulnerable and young people. In recent years, more and more young people have been going missing from London, only to be picked up along county lines by the police. That's if they're lucky. Some have been losing their lives to the associated violence, doled out as a form of control and a warning to others. Running county lines is a dangerous job, and yet so many young people continue to do it.

Among those missing from the community I'm visiting today are young girls, often from damaged and disorganized backgrounds, who have somehow become caught up in the drug trade more typically the preserve of young boys. Naturally, the community is worried about their children, and today's event has been planned so that helpless parents can share their experiences and address the issues. I have been invited in my capacity as a community nurse 'champion', having received the Mary Seacole Leadership Award, which is given to nurses and midwives for advocating for good health outcomes for minority communities and bringing about change.

With time to kill – a lull in my schedule, which happens rarely – I decide to pop into Westfield shopping centre, an imposing development that looms over this part of London, joining the surprising number of people who loiter in Britain's malls at any given time of day, seemingly with nowhere better to be. As I enter its hallowed halls, I check my phone and see that I have two missed calls, but they're numbers I don't recognize, so I switch my phone to silent and focus on taking a moment for myself.

But, of course, I am far from alone.

*

It's possible to lose yourself in the many wide walkways of Westfield, each lined with large shops spread over several floors. It is cavernous. Today, the footfall is heavy; every escalator and seating area, every restaurant and coffee shop is packed. The Black Friday sales have just been unleashed and everyone is here to make the most of the apparently generous price reductions. It's difficult to square this bustle of mindless activity with the warnings that the British economy is slowing down, that we are heading for recession, that the purse strings have never been tighter and more and more people are living below the poverty line. Here, dazzling billboards tempt us to buy, and then buy some more, whatever the credit card warnings might be saying. As I negotiate the meandering crowds, I can only assume that the ads are doing their job. But, between these expensively crafted adverts for various brands, I spot the occasional poster about 'mental health and loneliness during the festive season', and the smile on the face of the older woman pictured holding a cup of tea, looking out at the hectic crowds with a friendly gaze, warms my heart.

Despite our ever-swelling population, London is a lonely city, and the loneliness epidemic extends across the whole country. The festive season projects a false sense of togetherness – we are all having fun, aren't we? The truth is, beneath the gloss and sheen of it all, people are suffering from deeply felt anguish, depression and anxiety, often fuelled by the alcohol and drug use that underpins the British way of life, especially at Christmas. Suicide rates, particularly high among men and

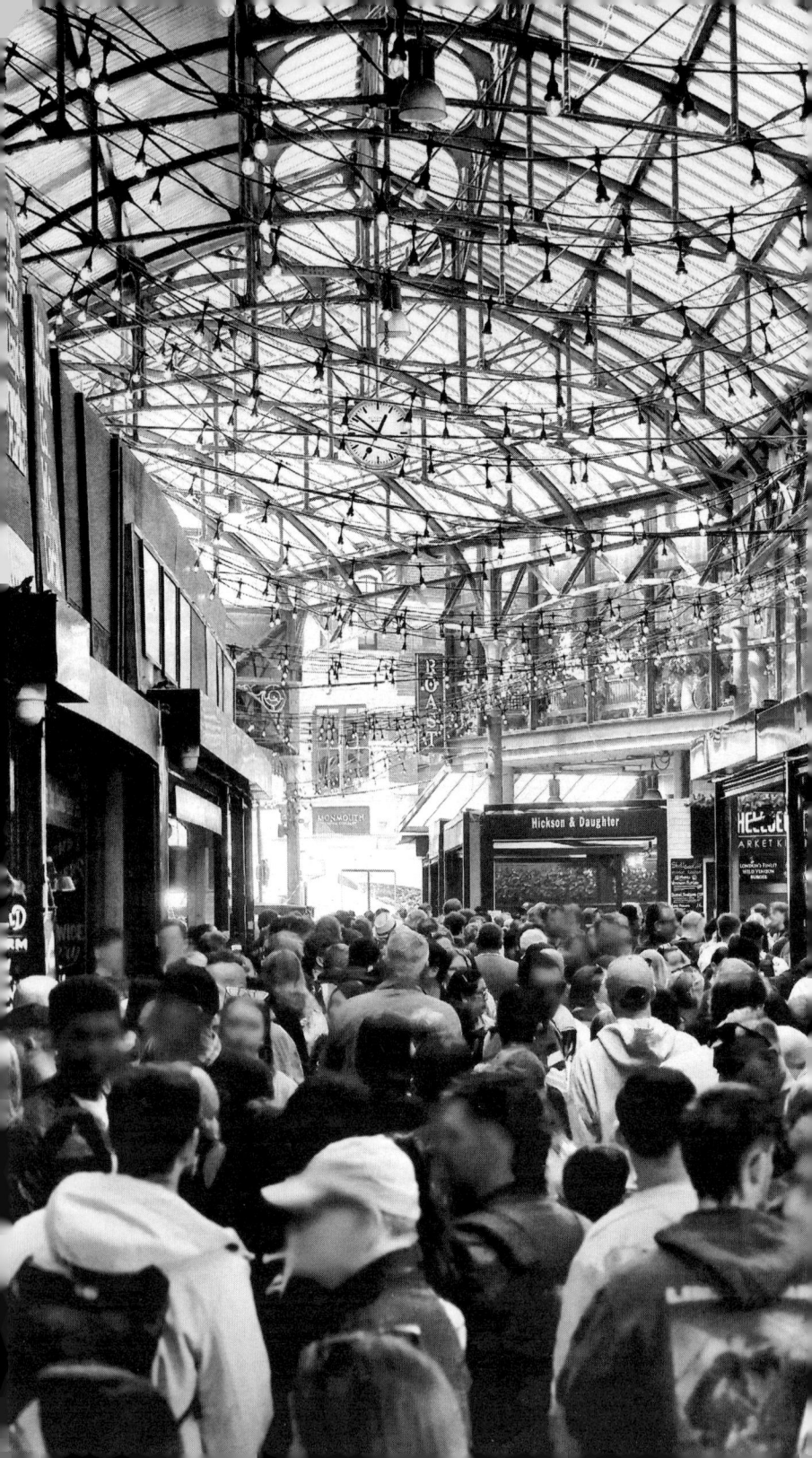

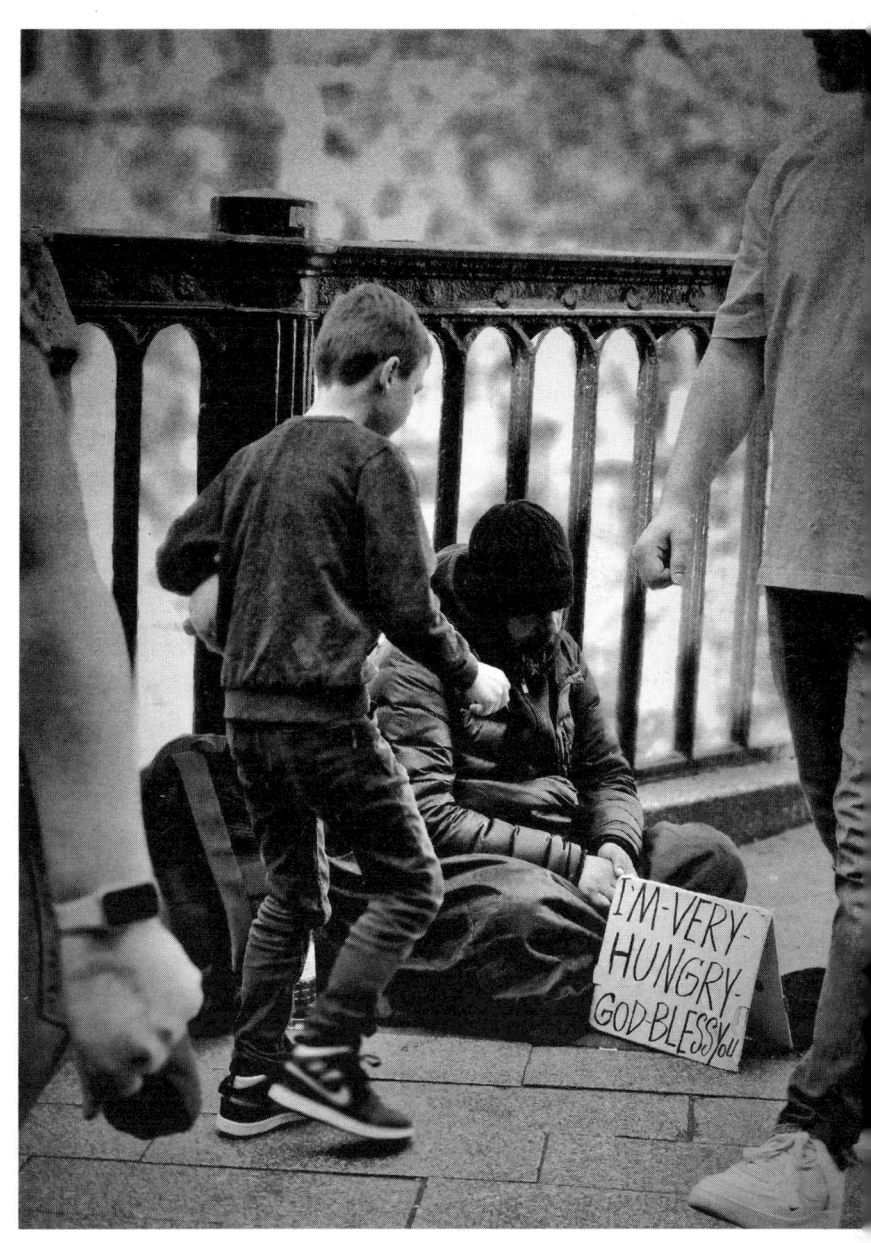

common across all age groups, are a largely unspoken blot on our society, and the festive period is a pinch point for many. Here in Stratford, beneath the bright lights of Westfield, you'd hardly know it – or at least it's easy enough to pretend the problem doesn't exist. Instead, mothers in flamboyant clothing defend their territory using their luxurious, outsize buggies. Men wearing custom-made suits and silk ties sip expensive coffee, their voices loud and confident over the hubbub of the shoppers.

A vibration in my pocket distracts me from my people-watching, but, by the time I find my phone, I've missed the call. I peer at the screen. This time, it's a number I know. It's Claudette.

*

Claudette's seventeen-year-old son Jevaun is one of my clients. I've been working with him for a while, now. Jevaun has been missing for five days and, while it's not the first time he's disappeared, it's the longest he has ever been gone. There is no sign of his whereabouts. In many ways, this latest development isn't at all surprising. There has been nothing linear about Jevaun's life, nothing straightforward. His past is complex, and his future is hanging in the balance.

Jevaun and Claudette were placed in the Stratford area after his safety became compromised in his own borough in west London. Having been pulled into gang activity, a drug debt had led to murder threats, with drug dealers knocking on Claudette's door looking for Jevaun. Naturally, she was terrified. Tensions escalated and the risk was assessed as very real, so Claudette was offered funded temporary accommodation elsewhere.

Managed housing moves between London boroughs are rare, but can become necessary, particularly where there are threats of murder. The risk becomes a significant safeguarding concern when children are involved, but these moves are by nature tricky, costly and disruptive for the families involved. Being uprooted is an experience that no one enjoys. And, while the problem may be further away, if only temporarily, it hasn't been resolved. The move just lessens the immediate risks. Besides, there is the new problem of young people joining or trespassing on another gang's territory, which can further escal-ate the risk to their safety.

Understandably, Claudette dithered at first because of the upheaval to their lives, but she soon realized it was the only way to improve Jevaun's safety and ensure her own. Despite their new location on the other side of town, the Gangs Unit has continued to support them, and I'm glad about that. Jevaun has been referred to me through his case worker, Bilal, who has been working with him for over a year and knows the family well.

Jevaun's early teens were troubled and he was referred to his local child and adolescent services by his school for behavioural problems, including hyperactivity and poor concentration. But, because his mother hadn't kept up the clinic appointments, the case had been closed before a full mental-health assessment could be carried out. Jevaun, with the help of his teachers, had turned to sport. He was a strong sprinter, a keen footballer and seemed to thrive in a boxing ring; his behavioural problems found an outlet in physical activity.

It was a good outcome, as we phrase it in mental-health circles. He seemed to settle for some time; he wasn't being picked up for petty crime, as he had been previously, and his friendships seemed positive and good natured. It appeared that he had turned a corner. But then one of his friends was fatally stabbed. Unsure how to process that trauma, Jevaun returned to the gang world through a group of young men who hung around his football club, and his friendships shifted. He was found in possession of drugs, and it was at that point of his downward spiral that he was referred to the Gangs Unit. Given everything Jevaun had been through, Bilal felt that he would benefit from some mental-health support.

Jevaun's work with Bilal over the past year had somewhat improved his behaviour, but he was never quite able to leave the streets behind. By the time the managed move was underway, despite best efforts, Jevaun's behaviour had progressed to the next level. He was smoking a lot of weed, which was out of character, and his bredren had changed once again – he was keeping the company of some deeply unsavoury characters, who were well known to the police. He seemed more angry, more brazen – he just didn't care. The exact circumstances in which he accumulated the drug debt that led to the death threats were vague, but, according to Bilal, there was no question that Jevaun had really messed up. We've recently learned that the amount owed is thought to be about £3,000.

Claudette, I know, has partially settled into the one-bedroom flat she's been allocated in Stratford. She misses her little comforts back in west London – the local bakery which sells Jamaican patties, and the street market, just a stone's throw away, with all its drama and noise. But, more than that, with the death threat continuing to hang over Jevaun, albeit at a distance, she remains emotionally unsettled.

Jevaun, we could all see, had settled less well. He seemed restless. There was no evidence that he had joined a new gang in Stratford or that his presence there had upset anyone, but the periods where he simply disappeared for a couple of days seemed to come around more often. Bilal wondered whether Jevaun may have got himself involved with county lines to make the money required to pay off his debt. It's a serious possibility.

As Claudette became more stressed about her son's behaviour, Bilal asked me to intensify my input.

It's a complex case, with a lot of moving parts and significant risk attached, which is why the allocation has fallen to Bilal. His own lived experience of youth delinquency means he's able to engage with his clients from a perspective and in a language that makes sense to them. Bilal, with his expertise in conflict management and training in cultural competency in youth violence, understands how individuals are shaped by their environment as well as their cultural values. He knows how much Jevaun loves his mother, and he is able to leverage this to ensure effective engagement and ultimately deliver positive outcomes, time and again. The combination of Bilal's street skills and my nursing skills has often meant that, together, we have been able to reach the most excluded cases with good results. I always feel it's a privilege to work alongside him.

But Jevaun's latest absence has given Bilal real cause for concern. This time, it feels different. The thinking is that a visit to Stratford will enable me to get a better sense of the place and the particular challenges that people in the community are facing.

Bilal has a rough idea of where Jevaun might be, thanks to his own intelligence network, but it's really only speculation at this point. Jevaun has periodically been texting Bilal from his burner phone – the cheap, 'unsmart' device favoured by people seeking as small a digital footprint as possible, and therefore popular among drug dealers. Not surprisingly, Jevaun isn't giving much away. Still, each time we hear from him there's a collective sigh of relief. A short-lived feeling of euphoria. He's alive, then. But we have no idea whether he's safe. And no idea when or if he's coming back.

If Bilal's county-lines theory is true, then Jevaun is definitely not safe.

'I don't think he's killed himself, Dorcas,' Bilal said to me in passing in the office, adding, 'I know you worry about suicide a lot.'

'With good reason, Bilal,' I replied.

Claudette has been worrying too.

*

When I accepted the referral to work with Jevaun, almost eight months before he was moved east, Bilal suggested that the best place to meet would be at the football club, which is wedged between a council estate, a major London park, and some unassuming local shops and lavish private homes in north London. The match was in its second half when Bilal and I approached the pitch to watch Jevaun play a little before having a chat with him. All the boys on the field were committed to the game, performing as best they could, while keeping half an eye on the coaches and possible scouts on the sidelines. Groups of younger schoolboys slowly joined to watch, still wearing school uniforms, playful with us and mimicking the players on the field, in awe. A group of young girls was hanging around on the baseline near one of the goals. They too, I could see, were hoping to be discovered.

My eyes were on the players scattered across the field. Energetic and fast, vocal and forceful, each signalled his readiness to have the ball and show off his skills. Bilal pointed out Jevaun to me. Wearing a red shirt with a number eleven on the back, he was moving with style and rhythm, confident in his footwork, strategic in his play. I could immediately see that he was a cut above the rest, full of potential – a north-west London boy trying to carve out a future in football that would take him as far away as possible from this fenced strip of Astroturf. I noted that there was no evidence of tension around the ground, but the gang members who had targeted Jevaun were unlikely to be active until a little later in the afternoon.

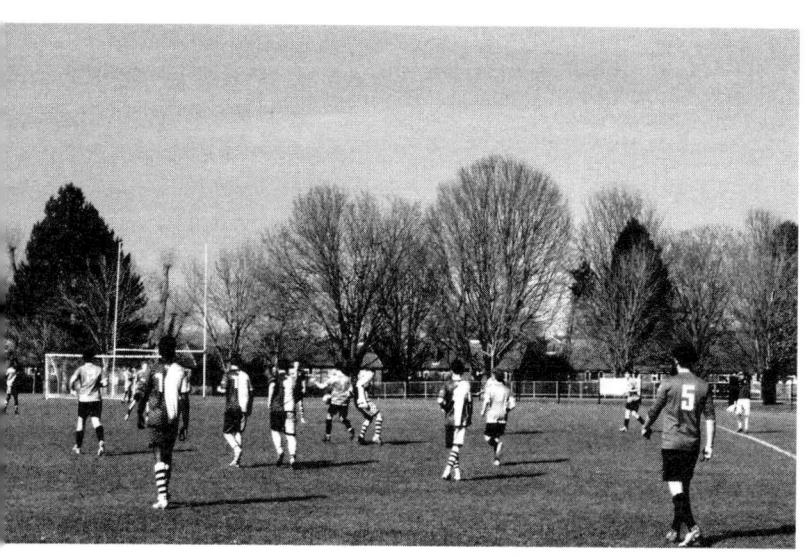

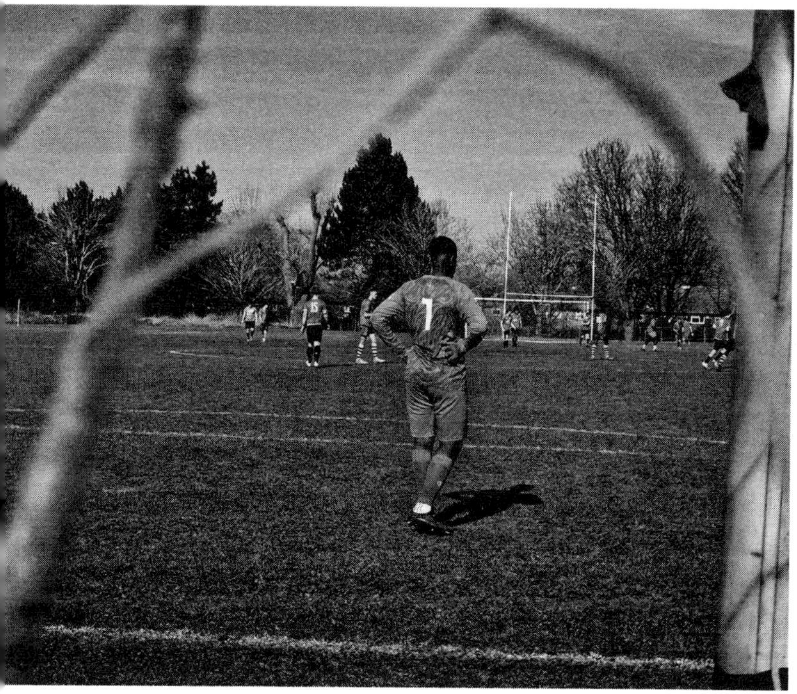

At the end of the game, Jevaun wandered over to us. Bilal briefly introduced me with all the usual awkwardness of any first meeting, and I did my best to put Jevaun at ease. In a short space of time that afternoon, we made a lot of progress. Jevaun said he was happy to meet with me and that he was willing to explore his mental-health issues, the post-traumatic stress he'd been experiencing following his friend's murder and the anger problems which were surfacing on and off the pitch. He told me he was also happy for me to meet with his mother, which I knew was going to be an essential part of his care. Then, with a small, apologetic smile, he slipped away in the direction of the girls. He looked back over his shoulder, as if asking us for the space to be a carefree teenager, and we were both pleased to honour the request, reassured that we would see him again soon.

Bilal watched him go with a grin on his face.

Back in the day, Bilal too had excelled at football, but at the time his life was being lived as much on the streets as on the football pitch. On a good day, football won his heart, and he would show up and play hard. But, for Bilal, there had been too many bad days.

Unlike Bilal, and despite his troubled background, Jevaun had continued to play football seriously after his GCSEs, joining a thriving club. He had enrolled into college, choosing to study for a diploma in sport, but his attendance was often poor. Playing football and the streets seemed more appealing than studying. But he had caught the eye of the club's coaches with his fast feet and vision on the pitch. They were looking to train him up so that he could coach the junior teams. For Jevaun, football was more than just a game, something to help him pass the time and stay fit. Football gave him happiness and freedom, away from all the negativity that otherwise surrounded him. From the moment he laced up his boots and stepped onto the pitch, adrenalin pumping, he found that life transformed into a realm of endless possibilities.

Claudette had told me about the first time Jevaun scored a goal for his new team, how he'd celebrated with his teammates, then searched for his mother on the sidelines, meeting her eyes, basking in her approval and acknowledging her hope for him. Football, they both knew, was a way to seal his future. *Their* future. It was football that had taught Jevaun the life skills of emotional regulation, anger management, discipline and compassion. He'd learned that his personal success on the pitch was for the greater good of the team, that victory was not about any individual.

Claudette was thrilled for her son. As she watched him grow and flourish, she allowed herself to envisage their lives beyond the council estate. She could see a job for him that would give them an entry into a world that offered greater freedom and more security. An income. A community. If Jevaun could find a career as a football coach, it could be their passport out of the inner-London tensions that stalked him. If only he could balance college and sport better, she thought. Focused on Jevaun's potential, she worked out that she could use sport as a trade-off. If Jevaun was well behaved and did everything that was asked of him, she would sometimes get tickets to see his beloved Manchester City play one of the London clubs. Mother and son learned to work together as a team.

But jealous talk about the opportunities that might allow Jevaun to move on and move away had rampaged through the streets. The west London gangs, who had given themselves jurisdiction over the football pitch where Jevaun trained, got wind of his possible elevation. How could Jevaun, the son of a single Jamaican mother, be better than them? Fuelled by envy, they set out to destroy his life, which is when Jevaun joined the gang, seeking protection, seeing no other way to stay safe.

The football club, fearful of escalating tensions among the players, the growing presence of gang members at the ground and the risk of the pitch becoming a battlefield, had reached out to local community leaders, who in turn had looked to the Gangs Unit for help.

Our job was to step in to dampen the tensions which threatened to erupt into something ugly, and keep Jevaun safe.

*

Jevaun and I caught up a few times after our introduction at the football pitch, meeting at a McDonald's in west London. I teased him about his unimaginative choice of venue. He teased me about asking so many questions about his health. But he obliged me, giving me the answers I needed as we carefully went through a PTSD questionnaire to explore his mood and sense of safety. He scored relatively well across the board, but seemed anxious. He was worried about money, he told me, alluding vaguely to buying something with a loan that he was now unable to pay back. My ears pricked up. Here was a young person from a relatively poor home but excelling in football, subject to seething jealousy around him and suddenly worried about owing some money. Now I too was worried.

But Jevaun didn't seem to be unduly concerned about his own safety; that wasn't his focus. He was more concerned about his mother, who had a long history of depression and anxiety, and was becoming increasingly stressed about the escalating risks to his wellbeing.

Then Jevaun went missing.

Children and adolescents who are exposed to youth violence and exploitation frequently go missing, for various reasons. Sometimes my work with them will slow down when they drop off the radar – after all, if they're not around, I can't work with them, and the onus of care moves on to other agencies, such as the police and social services. But sometimes the youth worker will ask me to stay on board, especially if they feel I can add value by offering parental support, and this is what has happened in Jevaun's case: my work shifting to support Claudette through the crisis so she can be in the best possible place to manage events, however they pan out.

As the days of Jevaun's absence tick on, I have been keeping abreast of the case, and have pivoted my work not only to Claudette, but to delivering community- and school-based mental-health and trauma workshops, raising awareness of youth violence and exploitation.

Both issues are a priority right across London and the office of the mayor of London has injected some much-needed money into tackling the problem. Quite simply, the more young people – and their parents and carers – understand about the dangers of gang activity, the better we can prevent a situation like Jevaun's arising. While public services are finally awake to the realities of county-lines activities and the associated violence, the communities from which young people are being recruited are still grappling with what it means for their vulnerable children.

*

My phone rings again and I catch it this time. Claudette. She sounds distressed.

'I still don't hear from him, you know,' she stammers.

I ask her if she has called the police yet, knowing full well that she'll struggle to make that call. Many parents feel this way. I know from Claudette that Jevaun's behaviour has drastically changed over recent months. The discipline and manners learned from his mother and on the football pitch have disappeared. Instead, he has been spending more time on his phone, trying to work out who is on his side and who isn't, who owes whom for something or other and who doesn't. He has been snappy and scared, but unable to admit to his fears. This turmoil of emotions has been expressed through anger and agitation. Weed is involved. Gangs are involved. So, no, Claudette doesn't dare call the police to report her son missing, despite her fears for his safety.

To involve the police is to open a can of worms. If Jevaun finds out that she has done so, he will hold it against her for the rest of their lives. It will also bring into sharp focus Jevaun's illegal activities, which Claudette would rather not make public, and perhaps not acknowledge even to herself. She certainly doesn't want to drive a wedge between herself and her son. She is caught painfully between a rock and a hard place. So, as well as supporting Jevaun through his trauma, I am here to support his mum with her mental-health challenges.

Even from a distance, I can feel Claudette's anxiety. I let her know that I can visit her tomorrow. Eager to share her burden, she immediately agrees.

*

I arrive at the community centre as people are beginning to stroll in, clustered in various family and friendship groups. Most are women, many of them young, their colourful dresses a welcome sight amid the sludgy shades of winter clothing. A few men from the community have turned out too. They are older, full of what they like to think of as wisdom about how, once upon a time, people used to respect their elders and, oh, how times have changed. It's an age-old story of social decay from generation to generation. And perhaps it's true.

I sit in one of the folding wooden chairs, several rows from the front, and slip my phone away, wanting to give this moment my full attention. But I am still thinking about Jevaun, hoping he is safe. I can't help but wonder if he is missing playing football. If he is missing his mother. Above all, I hope this episode is nothing more than another teenager pushing parental boundaries. I pray that he doesn't end up like the teenagers we are reflecting on this evening. I hope we have not lost another young person to knife crime.

The speeches start, the voices bouncing off the Victorian brick walls and filling the stark room. The opening words of each speaker are laden with formalities, with honours and acknowledgements and thanks offered to the various important members of the community who are here tonight. They're words that remind me of my volunteering days in countries like Tanzania and Myanmar, where cultural formalities have always had great value, propagating community connection and engagement. As speakers pause to search for what they want to say, or to struggle with their emotions, the respectful silence is occasionally punctured by the urgent sound of an ambulance or a police car racing through the streets outside. The city is always in a state of emergency.

Many voice their fears for the safety of their children. What they want, more than anything, is to keep their children alive and well. It doesn't seem like too much to ask. Then the mother of one of the deceased takes her place on the small makeshift stage. She talks about how he had been missing for more than a week when he reappeared unexpectedly, altered, stressed, his eyes haunted, his nights sleepless. In a trembling voice, she describes the morning of the day her seventeen-year-old son was murdered. There was, of course, nothing unusual about it. She had to wake him. He ate quickly, standing at the counter in the kitchen. The room is hushed as she haltingly walks us through what she is living, what she can't stop thinking about. The long and lonely dark hours of her son's wakefulness. The intense fear he must have experienced when it dawned on him that he was in extreme danger. The fatal stabbing. What had he felt? Then the arrival of the police on her doorstep. The overwhelming grief.

Then she poses a question that baffles us all: 'How does the law protect my son? Or your son? I know the police arrest them all the time, but what I don't know is how our young people are being protected?'

The young people who are present, mostly seated together towards the back of the room, huff and puff, muttering beneath their breath in agreement. They are fired up now, wrestling with the idea of imbalance between enforcement and protection, and how what happens out there on the streets is skewed towards the former. Who is looking out for them? The kids who have nothing to do with gangs, by far the great majority of them, are scared too.

A retired social worker speaks up somewhat in support of both the police and social services, stressing their role in protecting vulnerable children, saying how, in his time on the frontline, he saw some exemplary work. But his words in defence of these community services only make the room more agitated. It is not what people want to hear. It doesn't equate with their experiences of heavy-handed and ineffectual interventions.

To settle things down and take thoughts in another direction, I stand up to make a few appeasing points about the need to recognize the mental-health toll, not only on individuals, but on the community as a whole, and how important it is to harness community spirit for the protection of our children. It is, after all, why we are here tonight.

They are listening. Getting into my stride, I talk about the risk of sexual exploitation for girls, the risk of self-harm, of psychosis, depression and anxiety, using language that is palatable to the community. I emphasize that we must ensure people use the services that are available – understanding, too, that people may be sceptical about the very services they are being encouraged to access. I say that mental-health problems can cause us to think too much, that they can affect our sleep and our appetite, and that it's all too easy to become overwhelmed.

A middle-aged mother interrupts me and reminds us all how difficult it is to access a GP – the starting point for the specialized services that are out there. She asks, even if it's possible to get an appointment, would a GP really understand the worries she has for her children? I have to acknowledge that her concerns are valid. Before the managed move to east London I had tried to get Claudette to see her GP about her risk of hypertension and an increase in weight gain, which I was worried was affecting her mobility, but without much luck. The GP might well require Claudette to visit the surgery, but she had become too frightened to leave her house because of the escalating death threats Jevaun had received, some on her own doorstep. And so the vicious cycle is set in motion; these services are not designed with everyone in the community in mind.

The discussion continues around me, a series of questions with no real answers, words that are often full of sorrow, suffering and despair. But there is sometimes hope too. We all cling to that.

Afterwards, I make my way back to the Tube, the Christmas lights appearing more muted now.

*

I visit Claudette at her temporary home, a small flat nestled in a dark alleyway on a sprawling and densely populated estate. The London accent in this part of town is coarse and confident, I notice, the area offering a different kind of diversity from what I'm used to. Here, the old sits strikingly alongside the new; historic buildings that were battered by bombs during the Second World War have now been turned into expensive,

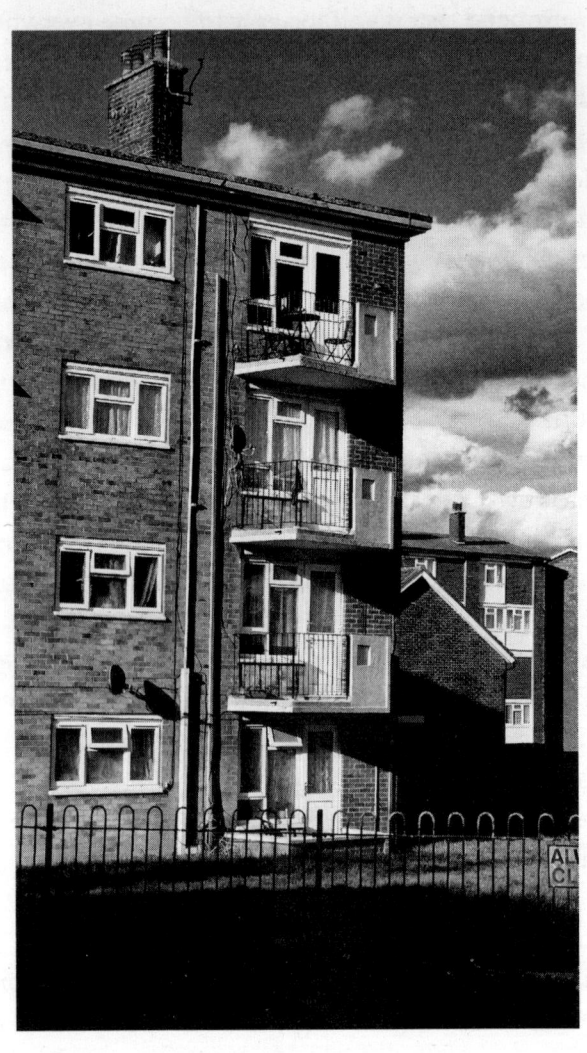

162 THE STREET CLINIC

light-filled penthouses. The London Olympics of 2012 brought with it big budgets and a national focus on an area of London that had long been forgotten and, essentially, abandoned. Now, pockets of high-end housing and retail development interact with areas of deep deprivation, and the long-term locals and more recent outsiders are brought together, a class divide rather than a racial divide.

Over the years I've been in the UK, I have learned that people make very quick assessments of where others fit in the British class system, informed by factors such as where we live, council estate or not, home owner or not; where we buy our coffee, *if* we buy coffee; how we present ourselves, from the shoes on our feet to the hair on our heads; our day-to-day behaviours in social settings and, of course, our accents. Youth violence and gang activity is similarly viewed through the lens of class. Society perceives that gangs are associated almost exclusively with people from minority groups, immigrants and the white working class, largely because they pay the highest price in mortality. And the media likes to make this into a story. What gets less coverage is that the drivers of youth violence are the affluent who buy and consume drugs in quantities. Here, as in so much of London, the two communities live cheek by jowl.

I sense the mood on the street change a little on the approach to Claudette's new home. It becomes edgier. But I'm aware that even the people who live here, on the fringes of the wealth located in the area's shiny new developments, hold themselves in high regard. The class hierarchy is alive and well. They can't help but compare themselves to harder, poorer estates, whether down south in Brixton or out east in Dagenham. There is a pecking order. Everyone, it seems, needs someone else to look down on. But what all parents are finally beginning to realize is that their children are just as vulnerable to youth violence and gangs as other people's children. No one is immune.

Outside the flat, I ignore the doorbell and instead, as I can see her, knock on Claudette's front window. She's startled and turns towards me. She has been looking out, caught up in the comings and goings of the estate, for who knows how long. Perhaps she is looking for Jevaun, hoping he might arrive home at any moment, as he normally would in happier times. I smile and I see recognition and something that looks like relief appear on her face. A few moments later, she comes to the door to greet me. She ushers me in and along the unlit hallway, where, despite the gloom, I can see that the walls are dirty and bare. It is entirely unlike her west London home, with its bright walls filled with family pictures taken in England and Jamaica.

We go into her kitchen, where the pungent odour of ackee and salt fish engulfs me. A stale bag of KFC is perched by the bin, not yet ready to be consigned to its final resting place. I get the sense that, with each passing day of Jevaun's disappearance, this space becomes more like a prison than a home.

Claudette moves carefully around the flat with a stick. She's only in her early forties, but her health is already compromised; the wear and tear on her body is a physical toll that only the poor pay. As we sit next to each other at the tiny kitchen table, I can see that she's worn out. This episode is the final straw. She fears the worst because she has seen too many parents bury their children and she has put on her best black dress to honour the dead too many times to count. And now, this time, it's her son.

She talks; I listen.

Claudette is practically gasping for air; she seems to be brewing a chest infection. As well as her physical health, her mental health is under pressure. Her motivation is low. Her sleep is erratic. Her voice is thin. My goal is to help her to manage her worries, improve her sleep patterns and consider improving her diet, and to encourage her to see a doctor for that awful chesty cough. But self-care of any kind feels like a tall order when the uncertainty of Jevaun's safety and well-being is weighing so heavily on her.

*

Tuesday mornings are busy for the team. We all try to be in the office, as it's when we share our plans for the week ahead, review intelligence emerging from the weekend and evaluate the effectiveness of our work, with our supervisors and the team at large. My mind is on Jevaun, but this morning I need to present an evaluation of the community-based workshops, which are currently being rolled out. I also need to brief the team on how the Newham community event went and invite discussion about whether we can draw any lessons from it. The demographics may be different from borough to borough, but the challenges are the same: each borough is engaged in a fierce battle with knife crime.

Bilal calls me mid-morning, while I'm queuing for tea in the canteen before my presentation. His voice sounds hollow. Something is very wrong. He is clearly worried and, immediately, I begin to worry too.

'Can we meet at the office at lunchtime?' he asks, the words pouring out in a rush. 'There's something I need your advice on.'

I try to probe him on what the issue might be, but he won't be drawn. He's determined to talk face to face.

My mind whirls. All I know for sure is that Jevaun is still missing. What I can't tell from Bilal's voice is whether the situation has deteriorated. Although I try to hold onto hope, it all feels pretty hopeless.

A text arrives from Bilal as I'm leaving the canteen. It says, *Room 5 at 12.45.*

Throughout my presentation, I'm on autopilot. I spend the next couple of hours thinking only of Jevaun, and dreading whatever it is Bilal has to say. It occurs to me that I haven't heard anything from Claudette and I take comfort in that.

Just before 12.45, I practically run to Room Five. It's chilly in there, the lights constantly flickering from dim to bright. The neglected facilities are a feature of our building, and yet another problem that remains unresolved in just about all our public-services offices. But the faulty heating and lighting is the least of our worries this afternoon.

Bilal takes out his phone and hands it to me, indicating that I press play on the film that he has pulled up.

It's a video of a young person being tortured. A group of teenagers and young adults, who might be in their early twenties, are holding down a young man dressed in dark clothes. His hands and feet are exposed, and they are being whipped with a what looks like a rubber string. The young man is lying on a scruffy mattress and appears to be intoxicated – whether from alcohol or drugs, it's impossible to tell. But he is sufficiently compos mentis to feel keenly what is happening to him. As the whip strikes his feet, his back arches dramatically, as though an electric shock has been driven through his body.

The light in the room is poor, which makes it difficult to identify the young person, and there is no sound, but Bilal tells me that most of the youth workers think this could be Jevaun.

We don't know where he's being held. It could be in the counties, or it could be closer to home. There are no clues. Perhaps he has refused to be recruited to county lines and the kingpins have chosen to demonstrate who has the real power. *You're going nowhere*, they're saying. *Think you can walk away from us? Think again.* Perhaps it's the drug debt. Perhaps it's a spill of information, a 'snitch', that has led to this retribution. Or maybe it's all of the above. We really don't know.

I stare at Bilal's phone screen as the brief video comes to an end, my heart in my mouth. I feel powerless. In modern-day

Britain, in one of the most affluent cities in the world, a young person – my client – is being tortured.

I eventually find my voice. 'Is that really Jevaun in the video?'

Even though Bilal has already told me the answer, I feel the need to ask again.

'We don't know for sure,' he says carefully. 'We're looking at how we can use the Modern Slavery Act to protect him.'

'But we have to find him first.'

He nods. We stand in silence for a moment.

'I think it's him,' Bilal eventually says. 'They want to destroy his chance to get away and do something worthwhile with his life. They're sending him a message.'

I think I agree with him, but I can't find any more words. I'm trying to orientate myself.

I have seen a lot in my lifetime. I have experienced a lot. I grew up on the fringes of the brutal apartheid system in South Africa, where Black Africans experienced systemic segregation, a cruel show of power by the white regime that was tortuous to live with.

During my school years in eastern Zimbabwe, I saw teachers whip children mercilessly for minor behavioural issues like lateness or swearing. Children were told to take their shirts off and were struck on their backs, or sometimes on their calves, using a rubber whip sliced from a broken tyre. The whipping, cruel and disproportionate to the so-called deviant behaviours, sent a strong message to the rest of the students. We lived and studied in fear.

I have spent time working for grassroots charities in the UK focused on safeguarding children from African backgrounds. I have worked with immigrants who have been victims of human trafficking, many of them from the eastern European belt and West Africa. I have worked with victims of female genital mutilation and with children and adolescents vulnerable to recruitment into extremism. I am familiar with the context of modern slavery, but never in my wildest imagination had I considered that torture could happen in London. This is new territory for me. Until now, it hadn't occurred to me that the Modern Slavery Act might be applicable to human trafficking and exploitation within county-lines gangs. I am baffled that we even have to consider the Modern Slavery Act in our thinking; it is a stark reminder of the gravity of the issues at stake here, in modern-day Britain. I realize I am still learning.

The idea that our young people might be subjected to this kind of treatment fills my mind with questions to which I don't have any answers. How can we keep our young people safe? What do we do with the trauma that this experience will bring about? How do we put in place the resources required for someone like Jevaun after this has happened to him? And if we don't strive to do everything we can to address and solve this problem, what kind of people are we? What kind of Britain do we want? And, the toughest question of all, what kind of person am I, if I can watch this film and do nothing about it?

*

In our weekly systemic therapy session, now run by Siobhan, a vibrant therapist with extensive experience working with multi-agency teams who manage complex health and social issues, we reflect as a team on the impact the video of Jevaun's torture has had on us personally as well as professionally. We also use the space to explore how we are coping with working with other complex families. Jevaun is just one of many difficult cases that the team is managing.

I start by talking about the anxiety I feel when young people go missing, how it escalates when *our* young people go missing, and the mental toll it takes to work with families whose prognosis is bleak and uncertain. I find that, once I start talking,

I can't stop – there is so much to say. I talk about the impact of our work – we all need to be reminded how vital it is. I talk about its humanness, how much our clients value our involvement. I also talk about how Jevaun always makes me laugh, and how the Jamaican patties in Newham may well taste better than ours in west London.

When I finally finish, Siobhan picks up and validates the work that we do as a unit. She sings our praises and I'm grateful for it. It's what I need to hear.

*

The next few days are full of information – some useful, some educational and some based on nothing but rumour and gossip. Crucially, we learn that Jevaun has finally returned home. He is bruised, exhausted and traumatized. And we learn that he doesn't want to talk about where he has been or what has happened to him. Even Bilal is unable to make any progress with him. Jevaun is determined to remain silent. Trauma, especially when so fresh, is always difficult to unpack. It's frustrating for us all, but I understand that Jevaun needs time. He is asking us for space. We have no option but to give it to him. He is alive, and we must be grateful for that.

Bilal informs me that Claudette has decided not to return to north-west London. She has asked the council to rehouse her in Luton or Bristol. Far-flung Cornwall is also in the mix. Anywhere but London. I understand this too. Although gangs are not just a problem for London – they are prevalent in many of the UK's major cities, and county-lines drugs have of course infiltrated the regions just beyond the capital – it makes sense for Claudette and Jevaun to get away, to have a fresh start. I'd like to sign off with them both, and I make various efforts to see Jevaun again, to review his mental health with him, but, for now at least, he has shut himself off from the world.

The involvement of our services in the case is soon over, but as a nurse I find that I need some sort of closure, so we discuss the case again, as a team, in our systemic therapy session. Siobhan reminds us that, while it may not feel like it, we did have an impact on Jevaun's life. A huge one. We planted the seeds of recovery from a mental-health perspective. We pursued and validated both Jevaun's and Claudette's experiences. We supported them through a transition in their lives. Our work has allowed Jevaun to see the alternatives available to him and, in the end, to make some positive choices about what might happen next. And that matters.

Still, it's hard to accept that Jevaun and Claudette have made a decision not to engage with us. That they have chosen to retreat into themselves. But perhaps that's no great surprise. They are, after all, a team.

7. Louise: The City

'Studies have found young women being targeted by male gang members who create the impression of romantic relationships before subjecting them to violence. Similar tactics, known as the "lover boy" method, are also used in human trafficking.'

THE STAIRCASE LEADING up to Louise's ninth-floor flat has an unexpectedly aromatic smell. A curry bubbling on a hob, perhaps, or a spaghetti bolognaise – I can't be sure. The odour is distracting, but it's something else that has really captured my attention and sent a shiver down my spine. Opposite the front doors of the flats, a tarnished metal railing is positioned on the edge of the walkway, the only thing between me and the treacherously steep drop down onto the street below. Despite years of working in council blocks as a community nurse, and being required to take rickety lifts or, more often, trudge up many flights of precariously steep stairs to people's homes, I still can't get used to heights.

It's early October. London health and housing agencies are on high alert following the dreadful fire that recently ripped through Grenfell Tower, the high-rise council block in west London, killing seventy-two people, many of them from immigrant communities. The survivors and their neighbours have found their voices, amplified by their local politicians and community leaders, and a strong sense of togetherness in grief and outrage has emerged. In light of this outpouring of emotions, many other council estates, in London and all around the country, have been having their flammable cladding removed and their structural soundness assessed. It's a welcome show of concern for people's safety – or, if I'm feeling more cynical, a piece of performative posturing intended to keep the many and loud disgruntled voices at bay. The jury is still out on that one. But the government has at least started to throw large sums of money at the crisis, as they tend to do in situations like this. It's typically reactive, not responsive, and this pattern of waiting for the worst to happen and only then doing something about it is nothing new. It may be too little and too late for some, but I have to welcome it.

Louise's council block, however, seems unaffected by the upheavals happening elsewhere. If there are any tensions between the council and its residents, they're not readily evident to a visitor's eyes; there is no improvement going on here, but life seems to be carrying on, regardless.

Mindful of the steep drop to one side, I cling to the wall and make my way carefully to Louise's flat. I find that my ears are almost popping at this altitude, but I can hear that the air is filled with music. Two of the flats on Louise's walkway are in competition to shatter not only my eardrums but all the windows too. The reggae is outdoing the jungle, and for a moment I'm lost in the lyrics of Peter Tosh. But it's outside Louise's front door that another sense takes over, the heavy smell of perfume almost engulfing me. Elizabeth Arden or Victoria's Secret, I can't quite make it out.

As I knock on the door, I can hear Louise's mother talking.

Charlotte's voice is always high-pitched, the tone shrill, and the volume more like shouting than speech.

'I can't find my mascara. Louise, have you taken my mascara again?'

'Mum, someone's at the door. It's probably Dorcas. We've got our session. And, no, I haven't taken your mascara.' I can hear the irritation in Louise's voice.

I have been working with Louise for a few weeks now. Having ended up in A & E after taking a minor overdose – eight paracetamol tablets – following the break-up of her last relationship, she was referred to her to local child and adolescent services, who then referred her case to me. She was seventeen, very nearly eighteen, at the time of the overdose. The transition from child and adolescent services to adult mental-health services should be seamless, but the reality is that many young people slip through the cracks. At eighteen, they lose some of their fast-track rights to secure and safe housing and health, and access to adult mental-health services can be sparse and complicated. There are additional risks with transient young people, Traveller families or families moving from borough to borough, city to city, or country to country.

Developmentally, this is a vulnerable time for young people, as they step into an exciting but sometimes bewildering adulthood. They are socially active. They are expanding their dreams. Some are moving on to higher education, some are seeking employment. Many are still vulnerable to exploitation and poor mental health.

Louise had swiftly found another boyfriend after recovering from the overdose. Having turned eighteen, she wanted to define herself not by the challenges of her earlier teen years but by the strength of her recovery. But her new boyfriend is known to be someone on the periphery of gang culture, which adds to Louise's vulnerability. It's this detail that has led to her being referred to our Gangs Unit. Eighteen is a significant legal age, but it's clear that Louise still needs to be looked after, and I am honoured to be part of a team supporting her. We've already had our first session at her home and have bonded well as nurse and client. We've set out our goals. Louise is clear that she wants more out of her life than she currently has; the issue is identifying what needs to change in order to get from here to where she wants to be.

Louise's relationship with her mother is as complicated as her taste in boyfriends, and perhaps reflects that particular problem; she is drawn to young men who offer her what she perceives to be protection and a sense of being looked after – something drastically missing from her home life. It was immediately apparent to me that Louise's relationship with her mother is a problem, a barrier preventing her from turning her life around.

Charlotte had Louise in difficult circumstances. She was in her early twenties when she fell pregnant by a friend of the family – no relation in blood, but close enough for him to have been regarded as her uncle. It was not a pregnancy she wanted to keep, but her strong Catholic faith left her no other option. Charlotte felt that her years of fun and perhaps even travels as a young woman were cut short by having Louise, a loss she's never processed therapeutically, raising her daughter amid these complex, unresolved issues.

As Louise has begun to blossom, Charlotte's been storming her daughter's stage in a desperate bid to draw attention to herself. A significant issue is that she's dating Bradley, a twenty-five-year-old who lives on a neighbouring estate. He's just a few years older than Louise, and the lines between parent and child have become even more blurred. The probability that Louise knows Bradley from her own friendship groups is pretty high, given the proximity of their homes, but she hasn't offered much about this in our initial sessions, and I haven't felt the need to probe into territory which lies outside our agreed work. She will tell me if she wants to.

Cheryl, our employment officer, is also working with Louise. Her job is to secure work, internships or apprenticeship programmes for young people who are vulnerable to exploitation. With Cheryl's help, Louise has found a job as a receptionist in an investment bank in central London. If she takes the job, she will be the first person in two generations of her family to break the cycle of living on benefits. I am thrilled for her, and expect Charlotte to support her daughter's efforts, but instead it's clear that she's consumed by jealousy. My work with Louise is to ensure that she keeps herself safe, away from the risk of another overdose or harming herself in any way. I'm here to support her emotionally as she transitions into her first professional role, and to help her to develop self-love in the absence of any meaningful parental love.

'I can't find my Louis V. handbag! Have you taken it again, Mum?' Louise shouts back over her shoulder as she opens the door to me. The accompanying eye roll is for my benefit.

'Yeah, I used it last night when I went out with Bradley,' Charlotte shouts pointedly, appearing in the hallway. She rolls her eyes even wider than Louise and we share a smile. 'Come in, Dor,' she says, squeezing past me and Louise and closing the front door behind me. 'Louise probably wants to talk to you about me and Bradley, this and that. She ain't happy about Bradley and all.'

Charlotte's pale skin is covered by a thick layer of foundation, beneath which her girlish freckles are still just visible. Her eyelids are artistically smeared with shadow, and black mascara clings to her long lashes. Her cheeks are sharply defined by blusher. From time to time, she flicks her beautiful bleached-blonde hair from her face.

Louise ushers me into the lounge, where there is a lingering smell of cannabis. The aged carpet is a gun-metal grey that sucks the life out of the room. Old family photographs hang haphazardly along the walls, and a sticker that optimistically says *You'll never walk alone* has been placed beneath a clock which ticks loudly. An ashtray overflows onto the worn coffee table and onto the floor below. But a few well-tended, vibrant plants are scattered around the space and bring some colour to the otherwise drab picture. I notice an ornate rosary hanging from a hook, as if in surrender.

I know that Louise is feeling the strain of living within the constraints of her mother's chaos while trying to build a life of her own. Her smile for me is small, her posture as she sits on the sofa is slumped, exhausted. This home environment isn't a suitable place for us to meet, but Louise says she prefers it, perhaps hopeful that her mother will see the effort she's making to mend her life. She's looking for a little recognition. But Charlotte is lost in a teenage-like infatuation and is riddled with self-doubt. She barely notices her daughter.

'I'm leaving soon, anyway,' Charlotte says from the doorway, 'so you can say all you like about Bradley and me.' There's a petulance to her voice. 'Dorcas, I'll drop you an email, OK?' she adds in my direction.

I nod. Charlotte has made something of an art of putting her feelings in email form, ever since social services became involved with her family. For Charlotte, email has become part necessary communication, part journal. Behind a computer or smartphone, she feels safe to release her emotions, frustrations and her truth. The mental load that should be worked out in therapy is instead being spilled, unstructured, onto the page. The heavy use of bold and capitals gives voice to her anger.

The front door slams shut.

*

There is a peace and clarity that reverberates through the flat the moment Charlotte departs. The family cat breaks the silence with a purr as she nestles into Louise, and I lean in closer too.

'How are you doing?' I ask quietly.

Louise's eyes are tired. 'I'm fine, I guess,' she whispers back, unconsciously pulling the sleeves of her top down over her arms, the fine lace doing its best to cover historic scars around both wrists, but failing. Her fresh Brazilian braids frame the light brown skin of her face. The overdose is a recent development, but Louise has been self-harming since she was in her early teens. Many of the cuts are superficial, most healing within days, and she has rarely sought medical attention for them. But the emotional wounds are deeper.

I allow a moment of silence, during which our shared space becomes more therapeutic; this is something Charlotte is not able to offer her daughter. Our parents and guardians are supposed to be our role models, but in the all too frequent absence of people to look up to and guide us, therapies can help us to make sense of the world, arming us with the tools we need not only to survive but to grow. They can help us to find our allies, people with whom we share common ground, and show us the power of the collective. It's uncomfortable that the collective often excludes those we most love. Having to look elsewhere for what should be readily available at home is painful. Louise is looking for her collective.

Applying some cognitive behavioural approaches, I attempt to unpack some of the anxieties that Louise is feeling about her situation and to address any issues that might be standing in the way of her moving forward. I allow her to vent.

'My mum makes a big deal about the whole Bradley thing. As though that's the real problem. To be honest with you, I don't really care.' She pauses, then adds, 'Well, I do care.'

Her teenage brain is trying to make sense of her emotions.

'The guy is twenty-five years old. My mum is well into her thirties. It's kind of awkward, to be honest. But, anyway...' She shrugs her shoulders. 'It's like we're twin sisters. Sometimes I could really do with her listening to my problems, but she won't stop to listen.'

I allow a prolonged silence to simmer, affording Louise the space to process this unsettling truth.

I am not sure how much Louise knows about how she was conceived and I am hesitant to step into those uncharted waters, and perhaps I don't need to. What matters is that Louise is losing respect for her mother at a time when she's struggling to make sense of her own emotional attachments.

Shifting gears, I support her in transitioning through her thought processes to focus on those relationships that are important to her and over which she has more control.

'How is it going with Nico?' I ask.

At the mention of his name, Louise fidgets in her seat and begins to smile – a full smile, this time. 'Oh, with Nico it's going alright, actually,' she says, the smile wide enough to reveal her light dimples. 'He has time for me, and he buys me lots of expensive presents. Like, lots of them,' she says eagerly. 'He bought me a new iPhone and the Louis V. bag. And sometimes he gives me free weed,' she adds excitedly.

My heart begins to beat faster. I know all too well that these are the kinds of gifts young men use to lure young girls into their lives. Once lured, they're then open to any level of exploitation. Given her existing vulnerability, Louise is at risk of mistaking those gifts for genuine love.

'To be honest,' she confides, 'I don't really see the point of taking the job that they offered me, because Nico can get me those kinds of things even without going to work.'

Her reasoning is alarming, but not surprising. It's a rationale that's consistent with her upbringing and the world around her, which has shown her lethargy, passivity and impulsivity. The people in her life have never placed any value in paid work, yet they place value in expensive goods and lavish lifestyles. Louise is caught between easy contentment and active independence. My task is to ensure her mental health is intact while also helping her to recognize that there is life – a good life – beyond the walls of this council flat.

'I'm here to support you,' I say gently to her.

She looks at me straight and says, 'What if they don't like me in that bank? What if they find out I self-harm? What if they find out I live on a rough council estate? What if I don't fit in? I am scared of that, Dorcas. It's easier just to run with Nico.'

I validate her feelings by reaching out and touching her shoulder, a gesture that offers reassurance and compassion. These are genuine fears. The prospect of transitioning into employment is causing her anxiety. I reassure her over a cup of coffee, which we cobble together in the tiny kitchen, and run through a simple 'Anxiety and Depression' questionnaire. Her score is average; given the circumstances, that's a good result.

We spend some time talking about music and the rise of TikTok, and, with the spotlight off her, Louise relaxes. But I know that, beneath the veneer, her challenges are a heavy weight on her shoulders. It's an accumulation of stress from living in an unstable home, poor self-esteem and emotional deprivation. The overdose isn't quite a suicide attempt, but it is a loud cry for help.

I feel the need to understand more about Louise's world, so I ask if she's happy for me to speak to her mum about how she perceives Louise's mental-health needs, and she agrees to this. How useful it will be, I'm not sure. I know I'll have to take what Charlotte says with a pinch of salt. Her thoughts are skewed towards her own personal needs and it's likely she'll try to hijack the agenda.

It's late afternoon by the time I leave. The walkway music is still pumping.

Safely back on ground level, I walk along the high street, which is buzzing. The local chippies are doing good business. Someone is chewing Somalian khat – a green herb long banned by the government as it can contribute to psychosis – and its mild smell hangs in the air. A burly traffic warden wearing hi-vis eyes up a white delivery van parked on a double yellow line. Schoolchildren hop on and off buses, their boisterous behaviour terrifying the elderly. Everyone calls this place home.

*

The next morning, I settle at my desk, sipping from a styrofoam cup of herbal tea. My inbox loads and I see that, as promised, I have an email from Charlotte. She has poured out her heart, but, as usual, she displaces any blame and outsources any parental responsibility. She is thrilled, she begins, that Louise is getting some mental-health support. But, instead of sticking with the agenda, she hijacks it, insisting that she too needs help with her mental health. *Not right now, though.* And I agree that the time isn't right. Charlotte goes on, telling me about Bradley and asking me to remind her daughter that she is a grown woman who can decide who she dates. *Age ain't nothing but a number*, she declares. In a rare moment of self-awareness, her last sentence reads: *Sometimes Louise doesn't understand that she is everything that I could never be and I wish her well.* The email is signed off, *Love Charlotte*, but I am left wondering what love has to do with it all.

It's an email bursting with emotional baggage. I'm not entirely surprised by it, but I still wish it read differently, that it was more supportive of Louise. It's disheartening for me and devastating for Louise that this is what she has to live with, but I am so proud of her for trying to stay afloat in a sea of emotional chaos.

I close the email and look for Cheryl. She wants to know about Louise's readiness to take up the offer of employment, and I'm keen to understand more about the banking environment and how Louise will be supported in her new workplace, a place that will inevitably feel completely alien to her. Cheryl's work is of great importance to the Gangs Unit. She's well connected to the London job market and is highly adept at persuading employers to take on young people who feel disfranchised. Her placements range from major supermarkets to banks, from IT to the film industry. Her criteria are clear: she takes on young people who are at risk of gang activity but who are ready to move on to employment and away from a world that threatens to destroy them.

Many of the young people Cheryl's assigned to are understandably drawn to her proposal. They like the idea of earning money legitimately and somewhat like the idea of having a structured day – although, they often struggle to get up in the morning, no matter how much they might want to. But some are frustrated by Cheryl's proposal because the salary on offer doesn't match the amount they can make from the streets. If they take the job, their income takes a hit.

Cheryl mostly helps young men to find employment, as they form the bulk of our caseload. But she also helps out young women, including Louise. Their trajectories can be very different. Girls who are transitioning from the streets to employment may struggle to settle into the new working environment due to challenges around poor social integration, reduced self-esteem and, sometimes, jealousy from other members of their cohort. But, in the workplace, they can also be further exposed to sexual exploitation, especially if they're placed in companies that already have a poor reputation for protecting vulnerable employees from abuse. Louise's vulnerability is a concern as she transitions into a job. We know that Charlotte has not necessarily modelled good relationships to her; indeed, Louise's history of relationships with young men has so far been difficult. Her risk of being sexually exploited within the typically male banking industry feels high. But I trust Cheryl to have assessed the risks thoroughly before placing her there.

Cheryl and I agree to meet Louise together to get a better sense of how she feels about starting the job at the bank. My feeling is that, although she's ambivalent, she's persuadable. We need to work out how we can both support her mental health and well-being so that she is in possession of sufficient coping mechanisms for dealing with her stress and anxiety. We need to make sure that Charlotte doesn't derail everything.

I also take the case to our systemic therapy session for discussion. As ever, Siobhan listens attentively to my concerns. She focuses on what is going well, underlining that it's remarkable we have got Louise to this juncture. We talk about Nico and the expensive gifts he has been showering her with, behaviour that reeks of gang involvement. A few of my fellow female team members and I joke about our own teenage years and how young men in our generation would attempt to woo us with ice-cream and a burger, if we were lucky. We can barely comprehend that this generation lures girls with Louis Vuitton bags and Nike trainers. But, then, the intentions of these young men are rather less benign.

Siobhan asks us some tough questions. What are the issues that are holding Louise and Charlotte back? How might their limiting beliefs about how the world works and the value of their place in it be overcome? And what is our role in supporting Louise to be able to think differently about her prospects? A fellow team member asks a poignant question: why are Louise and Charlotte both drawn to volatile and destructive young men? It opens up a discussion about parenting and boundaries. Someone affirms my own hypothesis and suggests that Charlotte might be trying to relive her own childhood through Louise, and by doing so is obstructing her daughter's chances in life.

The group's offering has me thinking deeply about how I might be able to support Louise that much more. Could it be that Louise doesn't feel worthy of a respectable job because those around her have never believed in her? To what extent does she value herself? It's heartening to hear Siobhan reflect on how Louise hasn't attempted another overdose or self-harmed since we got involved with her case. But this raises another concern: I'm worried that Louise might self-harm or overdose again if she feels that her mother, or Nico, are sabotaging this life-changing opportunity for her. All Siobhan can offer is the thought that, ultimately, any negative progress is not a reflection of our work, rather it reflects the difficult history and circumstances around the case. In other words, failure or poor outcomes are not reflective of our efforts. I need to hear that.

By the time I leave the session, I'm armed with more tools to help Louise manage her anxiety and build healthy boundaries with her mum. The group has reminded me that my primary work is with Louise. I agree with them wholly, but I can't help but feel as though we could do more for Charlotte. And if not, why not?

*

Louise has agreed to meet me and Cheryl, and in a high-street Starbucks.

I make my way there through the nearby antiques market, which is teeming with tourists and locals going about their business. A man plays the bagpipes, the humming, hypnotic sound providing an unlikely soundtrack as the buyers and sellers mingle among the overpriced goods on sale. An older white woman with colourful dreadlocks is draped in a vivid orange gown, offering Hare Krishna leaflets to passers-by. The smell of French crepes drifts through the air, making my mouth water.

Louise is running a few minutes late for our catch-up, and Cheryl is behind schedule too; travelling around London can be unpredictable. I fold myself into a cramped corner of the cafe, glad to have found a table, my hand wrapped around a steaming mug of coffee. When the door next opens, I look up to see a young man arriving with a young woman in tow. I blink twice. It's Nico and Louise.

Nico is striking. He is tall, athletic and perhaps of Greek or Italian heritage. From the way he moves, I can see that he is worldly and confident. And I can see why Louise has been drawn to him. Like a gentleman, he holds the door wide open so that she appears to glide, unimpeded, into the coffee shop. She's clearly conscious of being part of this attractive couple, and I'm not the only one who's looking at them. Louise is stunning, perfectly made up, hair painstakingly in place. Her cheeks glow warmly as she smiles up at Nico in thanks. If – and we do not know for sure – Nico is involved on the periphery of gang activity, he certainly doesn't look or behave like the young men I have worked with who are immersed in that world. But I know that these young men can also move smoothly through society, carefully diverting attention away from the less savoury elements of their character with their charm and style.

I'm surprised that Louise has brought Nico to our session, and without warning me. But I also understand why she needs the comfort of his presence. I decide to embrace it. After all, Nico is an important piece of the jigsaw and could be instrumental in persuading Louise to take up the job, which is due to start in less than a week. But I am not yet sure if I can rely on his allyship.

I stand up as they come towards me.

'Dorcas, this is Nico,' Louise says, her smile lighting up the cafe.

'Nice to meet you, Auntie,' Nico says, in a deep, resonant voice.

I appreciate this show of respect, which speaks to his values and perhaps his upbringing. It's a good start. I smile back at him and offer my warmest greeting.

There's intense eye contact between us; we are sizing each other up. For him, it's probably about trust. Who is this woman? What does she know about me? For me, it's about Louise's well-being and protection. For all our differences, we have in common that we both care for Louise, and that makes me hope that Nico can convince her to take the job. It's clear that he has influence over her. I can only hope that it's more positive than anything Charlotte has to offer.

As they sit down, Louise leaps in, as though she has read my mind: 'I've been talking to Nico about the job. He's kinda yeah and no about it, so I'm not sure, really.'

Acknowledging his power, Nico leans his folded arms on the table.

If this is going to work, I realize, I need to work with him, not against him.

'So, Louise has talked to you about this role she's about to start. We're really hoping she takes it up,' I say, smiling, keeping eye contact.

'Yeah, yeah, sounds good, Auntie,' he replies, without giving much away.

I'm wondering how his background might inform how much value, if any, he places on employment. 'Do either of your parents work?' I ask him.

'Yeah, yeah, course, man.' He seems surprised by the question. 'My mum works in an Italian restaurant not far from this

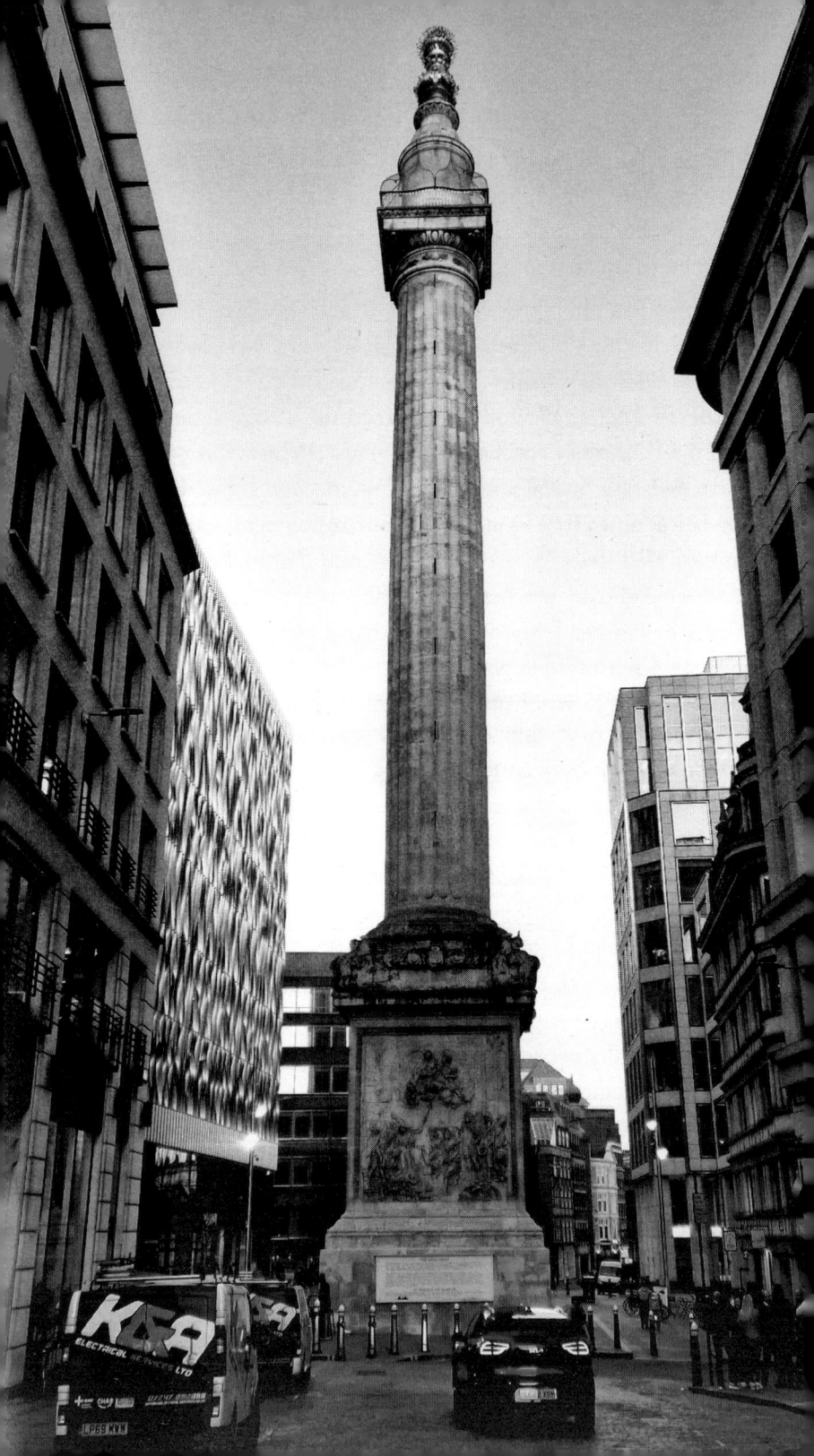

market, innit. And my dad works for the London Underground.'

Louise is smiling broadly as Nico talks about his parents, admiring how they appear to be role models to him. I don't have much to go on with what he has told me, but I'm also struck by the structure he appears to have in place in his own family. The question, then, is why on earth hasn't he found himself in formal employment too? Why do the streets have such a pull on him?

'I think Louise would be really good at that job she's been offered at the bank,' I say persuasively.

'Yeah, I know,' Nico agrees. 'As long as she doesn't take off with the next man in the bank, she'll be fine.'

And, with that, his insecurities are revealed.

'He's already got all sorts of stories about how it's going to be for me in that job,' Louise adds with a faint smile.

To take this job, Louise needs to convince Nico that she's not leaving him for someone else, someone 'better'.

'You know what they say?' I give him a friendly nudge on his elbow. 'If you love something, you have to let it go, and if it comes back to you, it was always yours. If it doesn't . . .' I stop there.

'I know, I know,' he tells me. He turns his full smile on Louise. 'I'm scared of losing her, innit.'

'But your dad doesn't lose your mum when she goes to work in the restaurant, does he?'

He can't argue with that simple logic.

'Louise really needs your support,' I continue. 'This is a scary step forward, and you can help her.'

'Like you're actually going to get up at six o'clock in the morning to go to work, though,' he says to her, filling the room with a burst of laughter. 'You can't smoke a joint and go to work the next day. How are you even going to do that?' He laughs again and leans across to hug her lightly.

'That's why Cheryl and I are here,' I say. 'With a little help, Louise will be fine.'

Louise has brought Nico along to hear that she has support.

'Right. Monday, I'll start the job, then.' Louise laughs loudly, the sound a mix of anxiety and excitement.

'Yeah. Right.' Nico's response is less enthusiastic.

Pushing his chair back and getting to his feet, he mumbles something about having to meet someone. He kisses Louise lightly on the forehead, gives me a polite nod, and we are left watching his departing back as he disappears out of the cafe and into the crowds.

Louise is at a junction. If she turns one way, she'll be leaning into Nico's insecurities and the job will disappear. But if she chooses the other direction, she'll take the job and work on building Nico's trust as she carves her own path.

Thinking hard, she brings her hands to her face.

I get up to grab an iced coffee for her and a mint tea for myself, giving her space to churn it over.

'Why can't I do both?' Louise asks when I get back to the table. 'Why can't I keep Nico and keep the job? Why do I have to choose?'

I don't pressure her for answers to these questions, simply acknowledging the difficulties that exist in managing the different areas of her life. For an adult, these are easy enough decisions to make, but they're tough for a young woman like Louise.

Cheryl will work on the fears that Louise has about settling into employment. I am more concerned with how Louise will manage the structure that the job requires: getting up early and clearing the toxicity from her mind each morning so that she can focus on the day ahead. Though her mental health seems intact at this point, I feel the need to equip her with the coping mechanisms that'll help her to deal with the changes happening around her and to her.

While we wait for Cheryl, we share some de-escalation techniques – ways in which Louise can manage encounters with her mum by acknowledging Charlotte's feelings while also defending her own position. We put a plan in place. Louise can contact me or Cheryl at any time if she feels vulnerable or unsafe within herself. She also has access to her manager at the bank, who she can lean on for support. Finally, I'm able to make a trade-off with Louise: if she works hard and gets paid, she can buy herself the very goods that Nico has been showering her with.

She is not alone in this. I feel confident that she understands that.

*

I get another unsettling email from Charlotte. The tone is high-pitched. She complains to me that, although Louise has been working for a few weeks now, she hasn't yet contributed to the household bills. But she has insisted that Bradley chips in, as he's spending so much time at their house. Tensions have escalated, but I am proud of Louise for standing up for herself.

I read on. Charlotte tells me that Louise has talked about self-harming but that she hasn't actually followed through. She suggests that I might want to check in with Louise to make sure she's OK. There's no suggestion that she has offered Louise any emotional support herself. Instead, she places the burden of care for her own daughter on the team working with her. I'm not surprised by this, but I am saddened.

She signs off in a way that reveals her own insecurities. She says she's happy Louise is working. *But just because she's the first person to work in our family for years, this doesn't make her any better than anyone else in the family.*

Whatever Charlotte's reasons for being in touch, I must take the risk of Louise self-harming seriously. I message her about meeting for a coffee near her office. She instantly responds and agrees to see me at a cafe in Liverpool Street Station, the heart of London's financial district.

The station has a fascinating history, being the site of the original Bethlehem Hospital, Britain's first mental-health institution. Founded in the mid-thirteenth century as a place of healing for sick paupers, at some point it began to take patients experiencing mental illness. 'Bethlehem' was contracted to 'Bethlem', and then 'Bedlam'. Today, the term 'bedlam' is synonymous with confusion and 'madness'. And, given how chaotic the station is during peak travel times, it seems fitting. As harried commuters push past me, I wonder how Louise is faring with the journey into work and back. It is not for everyone.

Louise is on time, which is respectful of our therapeutic relationship and, I hope, reflective of the new structure in her life. She is beaming as she takes a seat in the cafe.

'Not bad, huh?' she says, gesturing to her well-chosen outfit and placing her smart handbag on the empty chair next to her. Her braids are free-flowing down her suit jacket, and she gives them an occasional flick to position them. She is taking up her rightful space in one of London's wealthiest districts and is delighted with herself.

'I am so impressed with you!' I exclaim, laughing. 'How are you managing to get up in the morning when you were always still in your pyjamas at midday? Look at you!'

Over coffee, she tells me about the office environment, her colleagues on the reception desk, her supportive manager and the attentive Cheryl, who checks in on her regularly. All this is positive. Louise seems a bit aggrieved that Charlotte has been putting pressure on her to pay the bills, but I put it to Louise that it's entirely reasonable for her mum to ask her to contribute to the household expenses now that she's working. Coming from me, she seems to take it on board. I realize that neither

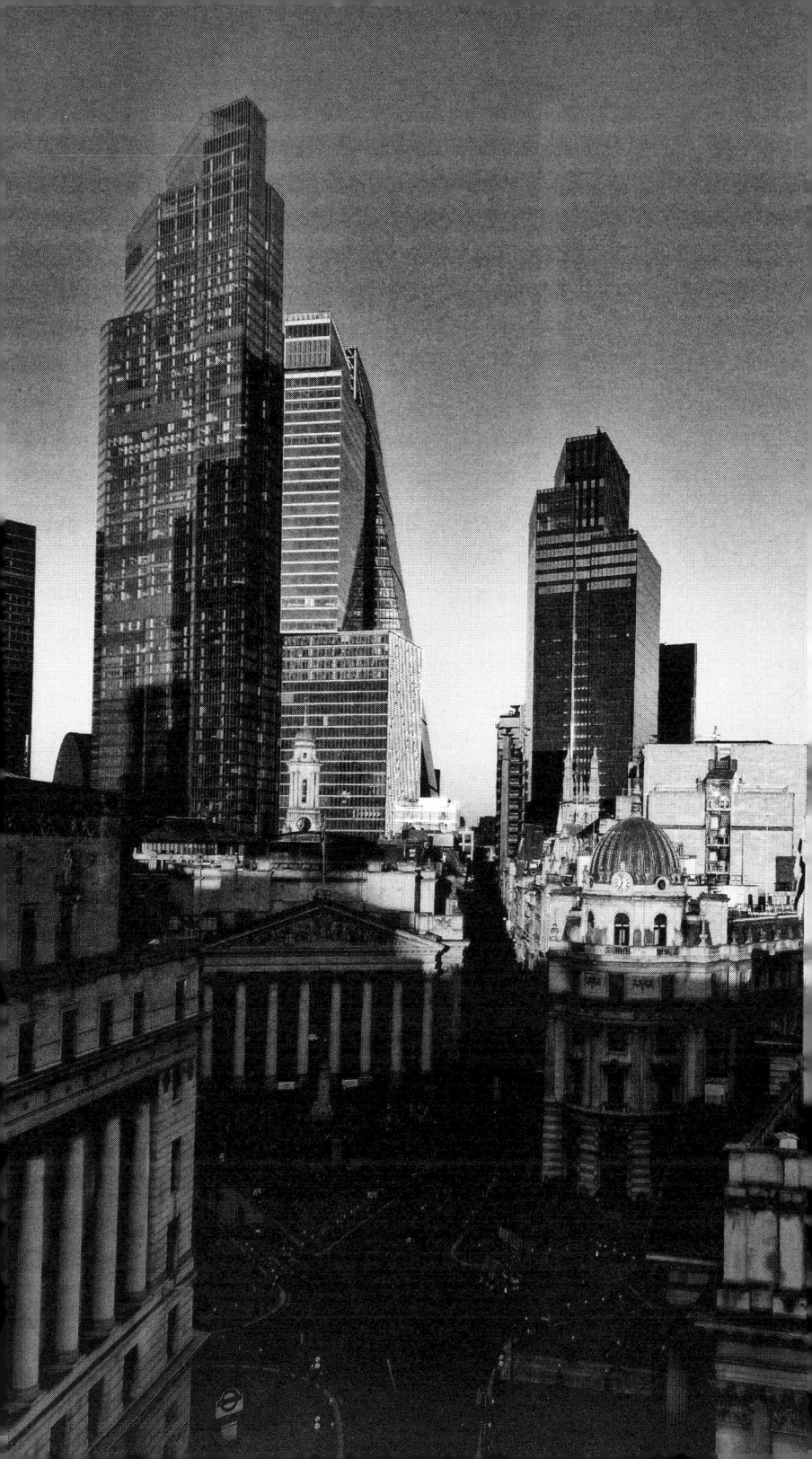

Louise nor Charlotte may have the financial management skills to work out how much she should or could contribute to the household. But that is beyond my control. My role here is to ensure that none of this causes unnecessary anxiety for Louise. I allow her the space to talk and I encourage her to speak with Cheryl about managing her household contributions.

Louise then shares that she's looking forward to one day having a place of her own. This time, I can't keep the surprise off my face. It's an ambition that demonstrates real growth and development. Louise is expanding her vision of what's possible for her in life. Perhaps the job and the people she's now encountering every day are helping her to see a world way beyond the walls of her council home.

The cafe is warm and Louise rolls up her sleeves, unwittingly revealing a fresh cut on her right wrist. It is superficial, but a cut nevertheless.

I come back to down to earth with a thud.

'Is everything OK?' I ask, leading her gaze to the mark.

Louise decides to ride it out. Even as I ask the question, I can see the defiant look that settles on her face and know that she will try to brush this off as just another minor self-harm cut, not necessarily triggered by anything remarkable, not necessarily meaningful. For some, self-harm can be a release of pain, a maladaptive coping mechanism that becomes habitual. In times of stress, we reach for the familiar. Louise has reverted to what she knows. Still, I probe. And it yields results.

'I broke up with Nico this weekend,' Louise eventually says flatly. 'I'm fine. Honestly, I'm fine. But it all got a bit much, to be honest.'

Louise is intentionally vague, guarding the details, perhaps so as not to alarm me and perhaps to safeguard her new job; she doesn't want to come across as unstable. I assure her that the companies taking in young people for employment on Cheryl's programme understand that mental health in the workplace is an issue they need to be able to manage, and they have measures in place to support their staff, especially young people like Louise who come from vulnerable backgrounds. Organizations and employers less understanding of how mental health can manifest in the workplace are less desirable to work for, and, these days, they can have trouble retaining their staff. The government has gone to some lengths to introduce policies that support mental health in the workplace, but there are challenges; poor mental health is costly to the employee, but also to an employer.

I suggest that Louise catches up with Cheryl to ensure this support is fully in place, but Louise is a step ahead of me. She has already texted Cheryl. She's taking charge of her own mental health. Despite my concerns, I can't help but feel proud of her.

I wonder what happened to Nico. Had he become intimidated by Louise, now that she was finding her way? Did Louise's new-found confidence conflict with his idea of what a girlfriend should be? Was it about control? Young men like Nico can exercise a degree of control over the streets, but they can't control the activities of London's financial district – its size, its affluence and influence may have made him feel small, may have chipped away at his ego. Emotional insecurity can lead to a quest for more control in the areas of life in which it's possible to secure it – and Louise will have been on the receiving end of this. I wonder for the first time if Nico too is filled with the kind of insecurities that have Charlotte in their grip.

Without me having to ask, Louise tells me that, after her job began, Nico continued to shower her with gifts, but he also became more domineering. It's as I thought. Nico was afraid that someone might lure Louise away from him, so he insisted on meeting her from work every day, controlling her movements and limiting her exposure to the wider world. Louise pushed back. She is shedding her skin, adjusting to a new reality, transitioning from the sheltered suburbs to the big city. I can see why those close to her who have never had such opportunities, much less seized them, might have difficulty supporting that.

I ask Louise if she needs extra support from me while she adjusts to her new life, but she is reluctant to engage in more therapy, which feels to her like a regressive step. The thought of going back to her old life is unthinkable. Despite this fresh wound, our case is concluding, the end goal achieved. Louise is on a new path; she may sometimes step off it, but she is moving forward. I want to keep holding onto her and keep protecting her, but it's time to let her go.

*

I take the case back to our systemic therapy session, where we talk about closure, what it means for us as workers and what it means for the vulnerable young people that we look after. Cheryl joins us. She speaks openly about how she feels to see Louise not only conquering her challenges but flourishing. She tells us about the differences she's observed between how young men adjust to the work environment compared to young women. Cheryl's experience is that young men are more hung up about the workplaces in which they are seen; they would rather not take up a supermarket role in case friends pop in and laugh at them. Girls are less fussed; they are open to all roles, including menial jobs. They just want to work, to earn, to have structure in their lives. I make the contribution that these issues are gendered, even in adulthood; many mothers will clean the filthiest toilets to ensure their children are housed and fed.

Other youth workers give examples of how they have found closure in their cases, whether because young people have moved on from the streets and got into the job market or because they have moved away from the areas of London we cover. A truth is emerging. Those who work with this vulnerable group invest so much emotional energy in the safety, development and wellbeing of their clients that walking away often requires them to seek their own closure. But it's elusive. A little piece of me will always be a part of Louise.

8. Hanad: The A & E Department

'One in three female and one in ten male gang members are considered at risk of suicide or self-harm.'

THE PSYCHIATRIC LIAISON TEAM at the hospital, to which I'm attached, is a service that has been commissioned to provide care to patients presenting to A & E in a mental-health crisis. We work in partnership with the general medicine NHS Trust, addressing both mental-health and physical-health problems. The psychiatric liaison team provides a twenty-four-hour service and is, by and large, nurse led, supported by a wider multidisciplinary team of psychiatrists, psychologists, drug and alcohol services, administrators, students and managers. As with any frontline service that provides such urgent, immediate and often lifesaving care, the team is invariably busy, and the relationship between the two NHS Trusts – psychiatry and general medicine – is one of war and peace. The atmosphere can be somewhat stressful and fraught.

The number of mental-health patients who have been fully assessed and are waiting for a bed is mounting. Some will be allocated beds that have become available long distances from their own homes, which will invariably pose challenges for their visitors to visit them. This then prompts a debate about who takes responsibility for the patient – whose patient are they? The general hospitals are irritated that there are so many mental-health patients waiting for beds, a situation which can test the core of the relationship between the two Trusts. But every crisis that presents here at the hospital provides an opportunity for us to think more innovatively about how we can keep patients safe while providing the best care.

Resourcing issues aside, in practical terms the service runs smoothly in nursing hands. When a patient with mental-health needs presents in A & E, the psychiatric liaison nurses receive a referral request. We screen it and, more often than not, we accept it. In line with policies and guidelines, we will see the patient within an hour of the referral. If the patient is already on the ward, we have a wider timeframe in which to respond. Once we have gathered as much history on the patient as possible, we then make our way from our psychiatric liaison offices to the main A & E department, a soothing walk which takes us past the canal.

I have always been drawn to this frontline, finding that I thrive in crisis management and problem solving. Today, my shift is focused on accident and emergency patients.

*

It's late Saturday evening as I walk into the busy A & E department. Like so many other NHS A & E departments all around the country, the space feels like a cross between a busy marketplace and a war zone. There's a steady murmur of voices, punctuated by the occasional angry shout or anguished cry as people seek and receive help for a variety of medical problems. Our frontline doors do not close – they never will. This is the business we signed up for. The paramedics keep rolling in new patient after new patient, while the walking wounded arrive under their own steam, until the waiting room, its six-bed

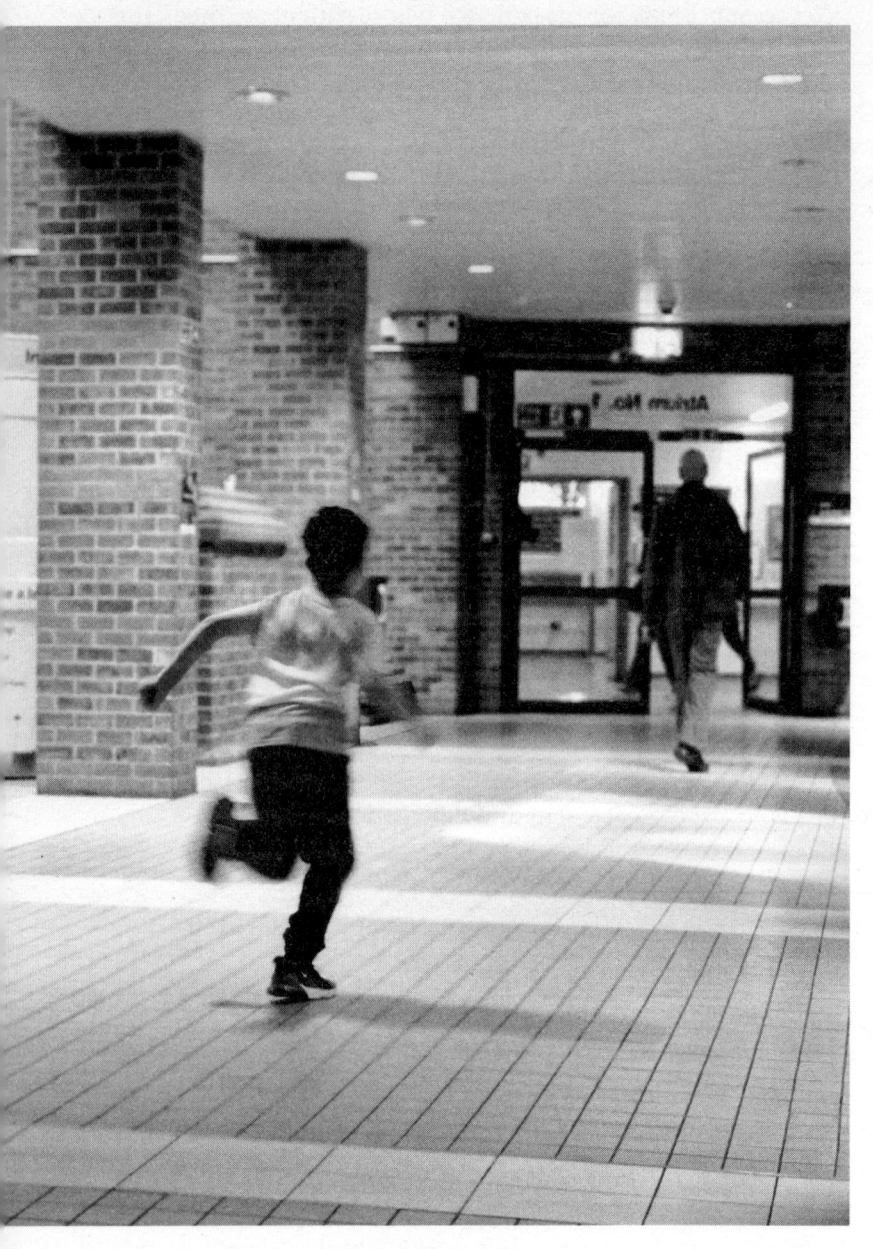

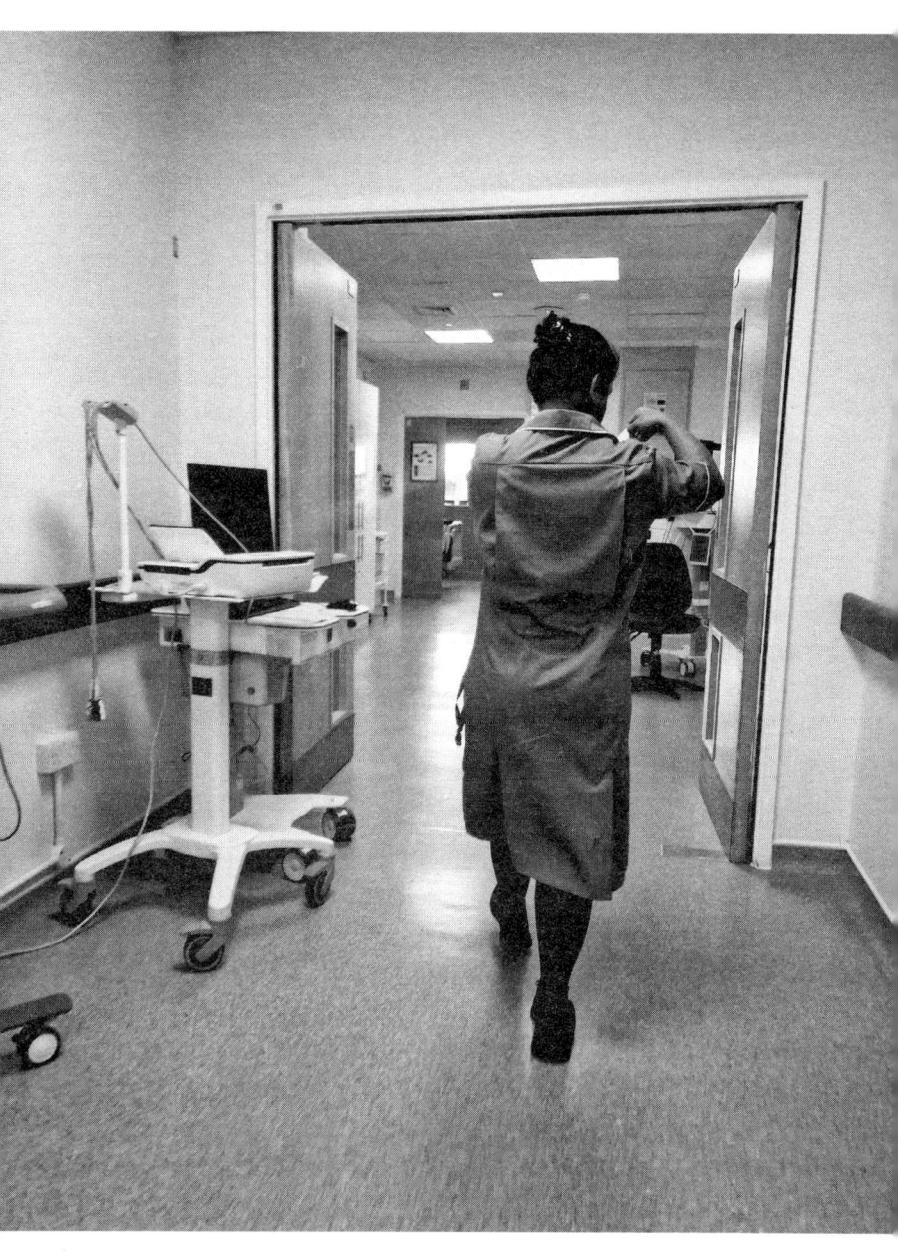

resuscitation – or resus – area and the department's cubicles are overflowing with patients waiting to be seen or waiting for investigations. The triage department is equally busy. It is a hectic time of day.

I walk past the paediatric department, which manages cases for patients below the age of eighteen. Some of the patients are teenagers presenting with knife wounds or wounds from fighting, self-harm or attempted suicide. We try and manage these in the majors adult section of the department, away from vulnerable small babies and worried parents. Staff wearing hospital scrubs run around in what is best described as organized chaos. But, while it may not look like it, the NHS is a well-oiled machine. It runs as smoothly as it possibly can, given the lack of resources.

How do we measure this 'lack of resources' in the NHS? When compared to countries that have next to nothing, and yet still somehow function, we have so much. It means our patients expect a lot from us; they have a right to demand a high-quality service. The NHS is a public resource, funded from the public purse. And we have the freedom to be a vocal society. The NHS has become highly politicized, with A & E departments functioning as the shop window of the healthcare system. Sometimes what's on view is attractive, and sometimes it is not.

In A & E, each person knows exactly what their role is, where they should be, when they should be there and what they should be doing. But the reality is there is such a lot to do, too few people to do it all and not enough hours in the day. It is, bluntly, gruelling work. If I could count the number of steps I've covered between the department of psychiatry and the A & E department over the years, they would amount to multiple marathons. Mile upon mile. Here and there. Back and forth. There's no medal to show for my efforts, but perhaps my lanyard is my badge of honour. I wear it with pride.

This evening, as ever, I have been summoned through a referral. As I approach the A & E department, I stop briefly to roll up my scrubs, which have sunk so low on my hips they're now helping to mop up the dirty rainwater which has washed in on winter clothing, squeaking soles and a sea of umbrellas. Around me, other nurses and doctors move with purpose along the corridors, ducking in and out of patients' cubicles. Their scrubs are colour-coded, a hierarchy invisible to the uncurious eye.

Wearing light-green scrubs, the junior doctors are particularly frantic. Society, we know, holds doctors in high esteem. Their credentials are valued, recognized accomplishments – the reward for many years of hard study. As our frontline medical investigators, they order bloods and analyse them intensely, in search of evidence and diagnosis and a solution to the problem. They then run their thinking by their seniors, hoping to have got it right. As yet, the juniors are too inexperienced to comfortably take on all the responsibility they're given, and yet it's theirs. Poorly paid, many still live at home with parents to make ends meet. They dig deep and find self-worth where they can; it is hard work but it is good work. I watch them flirt and fall in love within their ranks. They fill up the local bars and cafes in their time off; in their civilian clothes, they're unidentifiable as the people who help to keep us all well, but are prone to talking in raised, excitable voices about the cases they've seen. The horrors they've seen. It's a playfulness of character that's rarely offered an outlet because, ethically, we all continue to embody our professional roles even on our days off. It is difficult to leave the work behind.

My fellow nurses are also rushed, yet they move deftly around the department in their blue scrubs, elegantly coordinating care, moving patients from room to room and, when time allows, chatting to them, hearing about their lives – offering

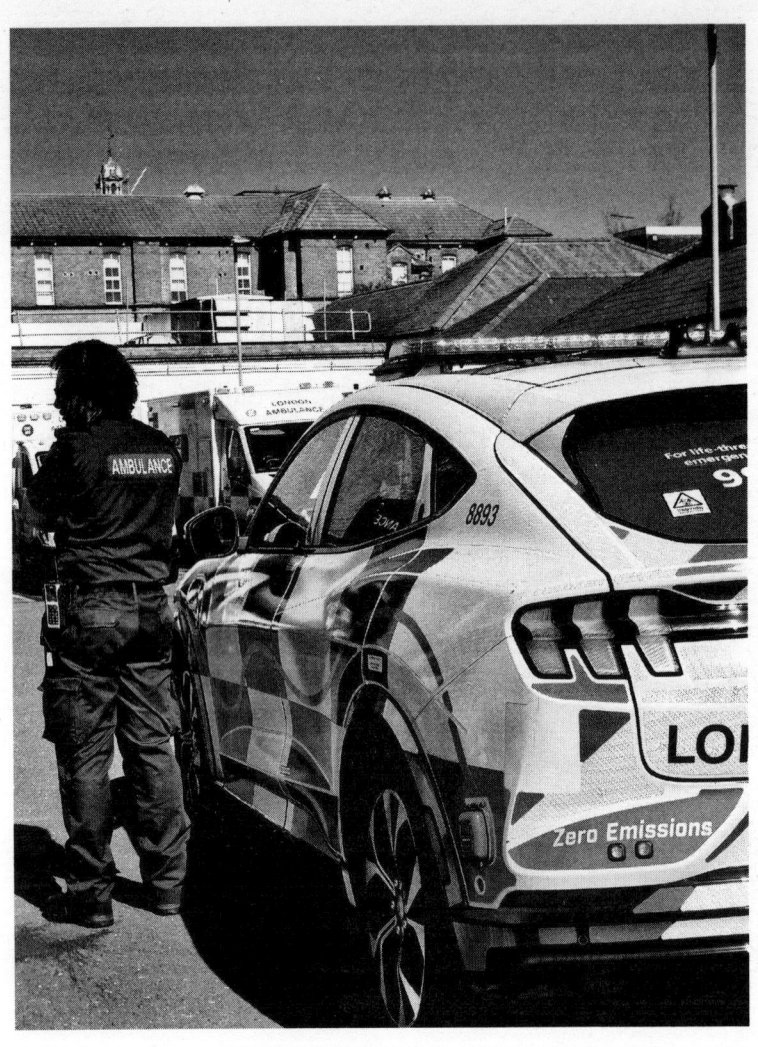

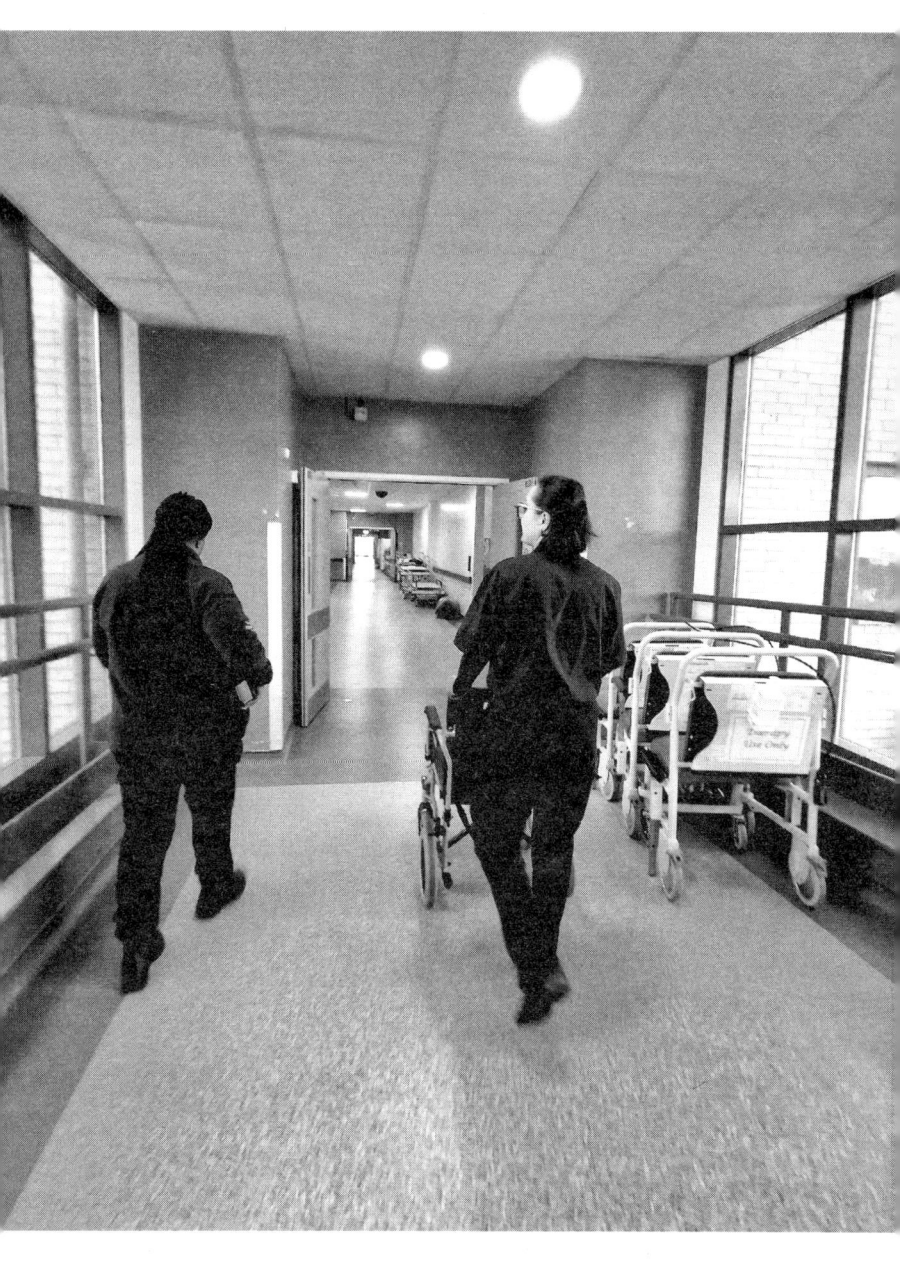

the little details of good care that matter so much but can get squeezed out when time is short.

A couple of cleaners are mopping floors that, before they can dry, are dirty again. It's a constant battle to keep the hospital clean, but they will never stop trying. And the porters come and go, gliding patients around on hospital beds and in wheelchairs, with polite dignity bestowed on each person, no matter who they are. I have always loved how compassionate and caring porters are with patients. I am constantly surprised that, however short the journey from one department to another, it seems to be just long enough to fill up with a conversation. They have such pride in what they do and, while they are sometimes loud as they go about their work, they are always full of joy. They lift everyone up with them.

The senior doctors wear purple and hover over everything. Calm, oozing competence and confidence, they are consulted on complex cases. They are the core decision makers. Their power is palpable and is felt throughout the entire department. I am enjoying that more and more of these senior doctors are of colour, many rocking hijabs, tattoos, braids or natural Afros. It's the ever-evolving face of London represented right here in our A & E department.

I take in my surroundings, even as I'm hurrying by.

My bleeper goes off again, startling me. It shouldn't – it has made the same rapid, high-pitched noise for many years now, and it's a sound I'm accustomed to. Still, I jump. I glance at the notification and increase my pace. As the double doors open to admit yet another patient, I catch a blast of cold air coming in from the canal and suck it down greedily. With it, the hospital odour I'm so familiar with floods my nostrils, a combination of blood, urine, boil-washed sheets and unwashed bodies that hangs heavily and permanently in the air, despite the best efforts of the cleaners and their powerful cleaning agents.

I navigate a path along the corridor, brushing past walls inexpertly dotted with pieces of art that are intended to help soothe the soul, the frames of which are tightly screwed to the wall to prevent anyone using them as a weapon against staff. I dodge trolleys and mops, the sad and the scared. I nod a quick greeting to a familiar face as we flash past each other. As another set of double doors slides open for me, I see that there are a few police stationed outside the cubicles of two or three of our patients. Healthcare and law enforcement often intersect in our department; there's nothing unusual about what I'm looking at.

But while the sight of these burly men in black is no surprise to me, their presence frightens some of our patients, especially the elderly, who are simply not used to a hospital space requiring such surveillance and security. Unfortunately, a police presence in A & E has become increasingly necessary over the years, as our patients can be aggressive. Some insult the staff verbally, others might be angrily racist, refusing to be seen by a nurse or doctor of colour. Occasionally physical violence rears its head, and has recently led to the death of a member of staff. That is something none of us will ever get used to.

With more and more of our patients presenting with drug-related problems, we are witnessing some particularly challenging behaviours. Of course, people of all ages and all backgrounds are taking drugs; London is a city obsessed with the consumption of drugs – for recreational use, to escape the daily grind, to feed a deep need that can't ever be sated – and its impact is keenly felt here in A & E. Caring for those affected by drugs has come to form a large part of my job as a psychiatric liaison nurse, because drugs such as MDMA, LSD, crystal meth, cocaine and cannabis can mimic psychosis and alter behaviour. The referral from triage might say 'a patient is behaving strangely' – this could mean a patient is talking to themselves, or threatening to throw themselves into the river, or compulsively shouting random words that threaten and scare the people around them. All of this can be interpreted as mental illness. And sometimes it is mental illness. But sometimes it is not. Patients must first sober up or get the drugs out of their system before any credible psychiatric assessment can take place. This means they will wait in A & E for many hours, until they are ready for a psychiatric assessment. They lie around in the corridors or slump across chairs, sometimes disturbing other patients. Their clinical management can be difficult and it's this that can cause friction between the two NHS Trusts.

My role as senior psychiatric liaison nurse is to gather as much history about the patient as possible, provide a comprehensive clinical assessment and formulate a diagnosis and care plan. A good-quality assessment will include medical, social and cultural needs, as well as giving consideration to any safeguarding issues. At the core of this care is the ability to provide a therapeutic environment for the patient in which they can feel safe enough to express their feelings, fears and needs, using an interpreter if necessary. Here, and in other A & E departments, nurses like me are tasked with nurturing these unwell patients back to something resembling wellness.

At its best, an NHS A & E department can offer the highest standard of care, comparable with anything available globally. At its worst, however, it can be a desperate and violent place, a place where patients sometimes die. The balancing act between care and safety is fragile. It's in this complicated space of love and hate, war and peace, recovery and decline that you'll find the most compassionate clinicians. Our ability to empathize and care in what is sometimes a confusing environment comes from a combination of dutiful service and deep altruism. And yet the system itself is unforgiving, with the administrative workload growing exponentially, meaning there's less time for the clinical practice we enjoy and are trained to do.

Despite the many challenges, I feel at home here. I love the camaraderie of the environment. And, although we are all exposed to dangers, there is a collective sense of looking out for each other that warms my nursing heart.

This evening, it is mainly drinkers filling the waiting area, slowly sobering up. Their injuries are mostly minor – lots of cuts and scrapes to the head, either from a fall or a brawl. They are all impatient to be seen, and the alcohol or its after-effects makes them irritable and sometimes physical. The odd elderly patient is visible through the curtains that circle each cubicle and offer a little privacy and the opportunity for confidentiality. With age, people learn to wait patiently, sometimes asking for a cup of tea that will take an age to appear, but they don't tend to complain. The young have a different relationship with time. I'd love to talk to these older patients about how the healthcare system has changed in their long lifetimes – surely it used to function so much better than this? – but every moment of my time is spoken for.

There's a friendly touch on my shoulder and, as I turn towards it, my colleague and friend Katriona, her Irish accent lingering on her tongue, whispers, 'I have another referral for you.' She smiles and playfully taps my headwrap, a fond gesture that speaks to our cultural connection. It's the sort of moment that keeps me going during a shift's long hours.

'Do you, now?' I ask, returning her smile, and we move to a quieter corner so that we can speak without being overheard.

'He really needs your help,' she tells me. 'He seems to be depressed and, when I asked if he's feeling suicidal, he was vague with his answer. I'm worried about him.'

I am keen to know more.

Katriona and I get on well, and our relationship helps us both to do our jobs better. It's a nurse–doctor friendship that has long gone beyond job titles and hierarchies, and certainly defies generational boundaries. She has talked to me about growing up in Dublin. Her mum is a nurse from Ghana, and she met Katriona's dad, who is Irish, when he was teaching English in her country. I'm fascinated by Katriona's experiences of growing up with mixed heritage in Ireland, which hasn't been easy, and she takes an interest in my global-health trips to Africa and Asia. She has told me that she took up various sports as a child to escape the racism she experienced and the constant feeling of being different in the society that she called home. She also speaks of Ireland's beautiful countryside and the walks she has done there, her love of nature and the outdoors stemming from the place where she grew up. In turn, I have shared with her my own experiences of racism while travelling solo in Vietnam and Australia, countries in which I had beautiful experiences but where these moments of race-based hostility threatened to derail me. I was attacked by locals on a beach in Vietnam because they believed that anyone with dark skin must be bewitched, and in Australia I was mistaken for an Aboriginal person without a ticket at the Sydney Opera House and harassed mercilessly by security guards in front of an almost entirely white audience who looked on without much care.

These incidents left their mark. But Katriona and I have also shared many stories about the joys of travel, which we're convinced has enabled us to be better clinicians: our experiences of being women of colour who dare to adventure; our ability to step back from the frontline of healthcare that we so love and step into a world of wonder has created space for our sprits just to be. Our worlds are bigger than the walls of this A & E department and, because of that, we are connected.

Today, when she smiles at me, I know she isn't just smiling about how pleased she is that I'm here to help with the referral. Having recently got engaged, Katriona is full of joy, and it's infectious. We huddle together conspiratorially. In our little bubble,

Katriona's fresh scent makes the department's odours, and the accompanying stench of fear and anxiety, simply disappear.

Katriona is glowing. She is in love, and it's almost tangible. Her engagement ring, a recent adornment to her left hand following a romantic holiday to the Seychelles, seems to light up the entire department, and she flashes it now with obvious pleasure as she flicks strands of hair from her brown face. I can't help but smile at how she dazzles, even in her dirty scrubs.

I lean into our professional friendship and listen.

'His name is Hanad,' she tells me. 'He's twenty-two years old. His depression is undiagnosed. It sounds like he has been involved in gangs. He was brought in by ambulance this evening, called by his mother and sister after he became very agitated and unpredictable.'

I nod. The referral aligns with my special interests; this is an opportunity for me to provide the best care possible for a patient who is among the most vulnerable in our communities.

'He has no history of mental illness, no physical health concerns,' Kat continues. 'He told me that he has been arrested several times by the police for petty crime and has spent time in police cells, but I felt he was minimizing his stories, as with all our gang-related patients. It's likely there is more to his history than we know. Either way, he looks quite vulnerable, to be honest. And, while I think the family are supporting as best they can, they look overwhelmed,' she concludes.

'Sure,' I say briskly. 'Let me look up his mental-health history and see what's showing. Then I'll go and see him.'

Kat smiles at me again, then puts her hand on my shoulder and gently gives it a squeeze.

'I want to hear more about the Seychelles,' I tell her, but I'm already starting to hurry away along the busy corridor in search of a computer.

Scanning the records, I discover that Hanad has had only

very brief contact with his GP for stress, nothing more. But what I've gleaned from speaking to Katriona is that Hanad's family say he's been acutely depressed since his cousin took his own life a few weeks ago. His cousin had got caught up with a crowd that was moving drugs from the city to the county lines, into the areas that surround inner London. He'd incurred a drug debt that he couldn't settle, and eventually his problems had come home to roost. The gang had threatened his family and, seeing no way out, he'd lain down on the rail tracks just moments before a fast train was due. He died a horrible death. The trauma of his actions has ripped through the streets and, for the kids who knew him, there has been little opportunity for outlet. In the aftermath, Hanad hasn't slept and has barely eaten. He has been smoking more cannabis than usual.

When a gang member takes their own life, it increases the risks for those who are left behind. They feel desperately trapped in their own situation, with no positive solutions available to them and little opportunity to express their emotions. A suicide will often leave wider gang members perplexed, anxious and, as with Hanad, depressed.

Put simply, Hanad doesn't know what to do with his grief.

*

Hanad has two families: the first is his bloodline, the mother and sister with whom he shares a home, and a wider family comprising aunts, uncles and cousins; and the second is the street family that his deceased cousin introduced him to and lured him into. At home with his blood family, with his father coming and going, the pressure is on Hanad to be the young patriarch. It is his job to guide and guard the women and to make decisions, as is the way within his patriarchal community. But London's streets aren't kind to young boys whose faces and accents don't fit. In a sink-or-swim situation, Hanad has chosen to swim. But his survival has required emerging as an aspiring kingpin among the local gangs.

He has exaggerated his 'street-ness' using skills gained while the family, as refugees from Somalia, lived for a couple of years in Amsterdam. In no time at all, he has found himself running drugs and committing petty crimes on someone else's well-established patch. It's territory that he doesn't fully understand. The violence that has ensued between gangs across areas of north and central London as territory is claimed and counter-claimed has left many young people injured, and now death has come knocking at his family's door.

There is nothing terribly unusual about Hanad's journey to London, which is home to many communities who have moved here from elsewhere in the world. It is human nature for people to seek a better life in a new place when it becomes difficult to live in their home country, for whatever reason. But immigrant communities are still highly stigmatized in the UK, often perceived as criminal, and what tends to be overlooked is how incredibly cohesive and coherent they are as a society.

In some ways, the generations that follow the first wave of immigration have it easier. They do not carry the hard expectations of assimilation that their parents faced. They can be themselves, and society is more tolerant of them. They are more likely to live between two worlds, simultaneously attuned to the culture and faith of their heritage while having a deep understanding of British culture and very much feeling a part of it. They might enjoy dancehall music, Afrobeat or traditional Middle Eastern and Far Eastern music, while also listening to UK garage, American rap and whatever chart-topping tunes are popular. Many will be bilingual, if not trilingual, which will give them an advantage in their education. Like Hanad and his sister, they will interpret for older members of their family who may speak less English.

Migration is about transitioning from one place to the other, and it can help to develop strengths and values that may be different from those of people native to a country. Those who migrate bring these qualities with them, whether they are validated by the society into which they're moving or not. Migrants who have been forced to leave their own countries due to conflict or wars are likely to have been exposed to violence, and the impact on their mental health can be immense. Yet they often build great resilience from that bed of trauma and tragedy.

Many of my patients have been exposed to trauma in their lives, which can mean they're not particularly fazed by the violence and exploitation they see on our streets, even when they're brought into contact with the very worst the streets have to offer. But, at the same time, their families are caring, involved and keen to do their utmost to keep their young people safe. Despite these attempts to support them, the young people I work with are often excluded from the mainstream and marginalized to the fringes of society. Young Black men are most likely to be profiled as drug dealers and as being dangerous to society, even when they're not. And, most of the time, they're not. On the contrary, they are quite vulnerable. The way they're depicted in the media and in fiction, however, seeps into the public consciousness, so that, when they do experience problems and struggle to find their way in life, there is often very little sympathy.

People see what they want to see, and hear the stories they want to hear. They shape the stereotype to fit their own narrative. The danger of listening to only one narrative is that we are less likely to appreciate the social and cultural fabric that holds these new communities together. The cohesion and sense of collectiveness the experience of migration can promote is something often lacking in our British society.

While many migrant groups face harrowing levels of discrimination and social stigma, they are not all over-represented in the mental-health system like young Black men are. Young Black men like Hanad are most likely to come to the attention of mental-health services via the police. Of the minority groups that I have nursed, the Black community is most likely to face challenges navigating the education, health and enforcement systems. They are most likely to be labelled as 'hard to reach'. It's my job to reach them.

Because of their behaviours – or, frequently, their perceived behaviours – young Black men are often treated with a heavy hand, bound in handcuffs, sprayed with tear gas and deemed to be dangerous and violent when suffering with mental-health issues. They are more likely to be sectioned and detained under the Mental Health Act, placed in mental-health facilities or prisons, sometimes for an indefinite time. We need to think about why this is and how we can do things differently and better.

While these young men can be resourceful in providing physical protection for each other, they are poor at addressing the emotional impact of the events happening to them and around them, such as bullying, stabbing, or suicides. It is, they find, preferable not to feel things too deeply. But it is not easy to push these feelings down.

*

As a clinician, I need to gain Hanad's trust as quickly as possible. Trust, or the lack of it, is a significant factor for young people who are exposed to youth violence and gang exploitation. Put simply, many of them do not trust the authorities – and with reason. I need Hanad to feel safe in our clinical environment. I need him to talk to me.

Alone with him in a small walled cubicle, I let Hanad know

that I have discussed his case with my colleague, Katriona. Using language and an approach that I hope will make him feel comfortable, I tell him that I already know a few things about his history and the reasons he has ended up in our A & E department today. He seems to appreciate being seen for who he really is and what he is going through. Young people often disengage abruptly with professionals who use complicated words they're unable to make sense of. Once the medical or psychiatric language is diluted and is palatable to them, there is more chance that they'll engage. Being so familiar with the language used on the street, it's easy for me to adapt for these assessments.

As we start to talk, I see Hanad's shoulders drop a little. He seems reassured when I say that I've done a lot of work with young people presenting with a range of traumatic experiences, here in London and also in Africa, where both our families are from.

Our families. It's important to make this point, that we are alike, that we share common ground, and I look for eye contact with him as he paces around the confined space.

In a further attempt to put him at ease, I ask about his experiences in the Netherlands, and about football, which I know he loves, and then about his friends. But he is still too stressed and anxious to engage in light conversation.

He stops me.

'Miss, my cousin killed himself,' he interjects. 'The guy killed himself. It should never have got that far.'

He looks at me properly, for the first time. Three short sentences spill out.

'The train ran over him. He killed himself. It's haram in my religion.'

This is my cue to open up the therapeutic space for him to express his feelings. I allow for a moment of silence, and he fills it, taking this opportunity to let it all out, to weep and grieve openly. Here, with me, he doesn't have to play the strong patriarch or the tough man on the streets. He clasps his face in his hands, his slender fingers trembling as he searches for answers. He punctures the silence with a shallow scream, then cries without shame, a deep, rasping sound that forces its way up from the back of his throat and is full of fear.

For young vulnerable men caught up in the gang world, fear can manifest in many ways. There is a fear of admitting to themselves that they are scared, and their tightly held fear is often managed through substance misuse. They're also afraid of appearing fearful with their friends, and particularly in front of their enemies, so their behaviour is carefully managed so as not to reflect that fear. It might be expressed as violence towards others, sometimes towards women, who are easy targets in their social circles. Fear might be expressed through mania, through erratic and chaotic behaviours that puzzle society but make complete sense to them. There is enormous clinical value in providing a therapeutic space for these young people to express their fear, and an encounter with a mental-health specialist may well be the only chance they will have to let it out.

Hanad's fear has manifested in depression. His sleep has been disturbed and he has been completely distracted. He lacks interest in the world around him and the motivation to do anything, and, as he sits with his head in his hands, he mutters that he would be better off away from this world, a world which is closing in on him. Caught up in the drug debt that led to his cousin's death, with his street soldiers disappearing, either to prison or to an early grave, he is alone. Hanad is deeply vulnerable.

I ask him if he has had any thoughts of ending his life. He doesn't reply.

*

The A & E department alarm erupts, a sharp and persistent high-pitched noise which cuts through the intensity of the moment. A commotion has been building up outside our cubicle and has developed into a major incident. Through the frosted glass pane, I can see police bustling around a man who is most likely a patient. He's screaming, 'Get those fucking handcuffs off me, mate! If you don't let me go, I'll beat the shit out of everyone in here!'

I pause. I do not open the door. I know better than to let the wave of violence outside wash into my safe space with a vulnerable patient. I look at Hanad to reassure him. He seems worried, although not by the screaming man. The presence of police right outside our cubicle has startled him, reminding him of the many times when it has been him running from the officers or being manhandled and arrested. I know he's feeling trapped here in the A & E department; young men who are involved in youth violence don't do well with all the waiting that goes on in clinical environments, and the loss of control that comes with it. In a place where other people have come to seek sanctuary, Hanad's sense of safety is threatened. The absence of his bredren, who would otherwise look out for him, scares him. All too often, it means that, no sooner than they have checked in, boys like Hanad just up and leave, uncared for.

The noise outside dies down; between them, the police and security guards have managed the situation. Job done, they depart – until next time.

Kat passes through, partly to check on progress, but also to check on my safety. For most people, it's impossible to imagine not feeling safe at work, but it's hardwired into the team here to constantly check on each other. An injury to one is an injury to us all. I smile at her. All is well, I confirm with my eyes. I am safe with Hanad. But I'm not yet finished with him. My senior nursing colleagues are looking to me to make a decision on his care and I'm not able to do that until we've had a bigger conversation.

*

Hanad is calmer now. He has stopped pacing and appears lost in thought. I need to know what he's thinking and to be sure that he feels safe within himself, that he has no plans to harm himself – or, indeed, anyone else. Eventually, after a prolonged silence, he tells me that he has thought about it, though he goes on to say that he doesn't think he would ever actually kill himself. But I can see that the thoughts are present and are distressing him.

I have spent a lot of time thinking about how some people who have lost members of their family are pushing back against the phrase 'committed suicide'. They argue that the word 'committed' is problematic, because their loved ones are not criminals, they didn't commit a crime and they shouldn't be judged or blamed for taking their own lives. Across society, there are differing views on suicide, and I wonder what those views say about our basic humanity. I think about my school friend who took his own life while waiting for his exam results. He was just sixteen years old and life was already too much for him. His unnecessary death is partly why I'm here today.

Working on the NHS frontline, I am very aware that many people struggle with their mental health. We live in a society that expects so much of us all, including the weak and the fragile. We are expected to soldier on, sometimes in silence. Men generally kill themselves more than women do, and a man who kills himself is often viewed as less manly than one who carries on with life stoically. Yet the man who's able to keep going may also be suffering deeply with depression or anxiety, it's just not as visible to those around him. Hanad's religion forbids suicide or the thought of taking one's own life, and yet his is a culture where there is no meaningful outlet for a man to express vulnerability.

In liaison psychiatry, we place value on appreciating the individual patient as part of a wider family or community. This has been drilled into me by mentors and supervisors who, through their teaching and leadership, have supported me to improve the quality of nursing care that I am able to provide to patients. These standards have further been reinforced by my work with communities in Asia and Africa. The concept of ubuntu is a southern African philosophy that views the individual within the context of the collective. It says, 'It takes a village to raise a child' and 'I am because we are.' Ubuntu recognizes that individuals like Hanad come from a wider network that holds its values, beliefs and wisdom close and draws from wells of ancient knowledge and courage, especially when challenged.

Hanad is part of a wider community. He has friends he has made on the streets – friends whom he holds in high regard, but who can't support him now – and he has his home community of his mother and sister. I know that, in order to fully understand Hanad, I need to speak to his sister and mother. In liaison psychiatry, we value any collateral information the family can share with us; however, the patient must give consent for us to speak to their family members – this is important. When we're able to have them, these conversations often give a clearer sense of how the patient's history informs their current vulnerabilities, the risks they're facing and the support we can offer in terms of a discharge plan, where appropriate.

Aware of just how vulnerable he is, Hanad grants me permission to discuss his care with the two women in his life.

*

'As-salamu alaykum.'

I bow my head in recognition of the family's cultural practices as I greet Hanad's mother and sister in the relatives' room, where they have been waiting patiently. I look first to his mother, her fearful eyes brimming with tears, which she wipes away with a corner of her hijab. Hanad's sister looks a few years older than him and wears a bright red hijab beneath a long black coat. Tall and elegant, her high cheekbones appear flushed, her modest make-up emphasizing her natural beauty. Her effortless poise confers authority as she stands between me and her mother, translating from English to Somali so that her mother stays up to speed with the proceedings.

Hanad's mother is distressed and anxious. Most mothers in our A & E department are, given that they're usually here at a time of crisis. I need to create a therapeutic space built on compassion and empathy so that we can talk. I gently ask about their family's background. Much of what they tell me I already know, of course, but it's a subject that helps to build trust between us. As Hanad's mum shares some of their story, she begins to relax. I learn that Hanad's family fled the war in Somalia and first moved to neighbouring Kenya, where Hanad and his sister were both born. They lived in a refugee centre there for some years, then moved to the Netherlands, where they settled for a time. Later, they came to London, their preferred final destination, as they have relatives here. Hanad's father travels between the Netherlands and the UK. In need of a proxy head of his London household, Hanad was placed in this position from a young age. It's a big ask of such a young person.

Hanad's sister takes charge of the conversation. Confident and assertive, she navigates between her mother's feelings and her brother's needs, switching between Somali and English, holding her mother's hand all the while. Not for the first time, I am looking at a young woman who has grown up in a sometimes troubled environment, who necessarily acts as a support system for the wider family. These extraordinary girls are highly

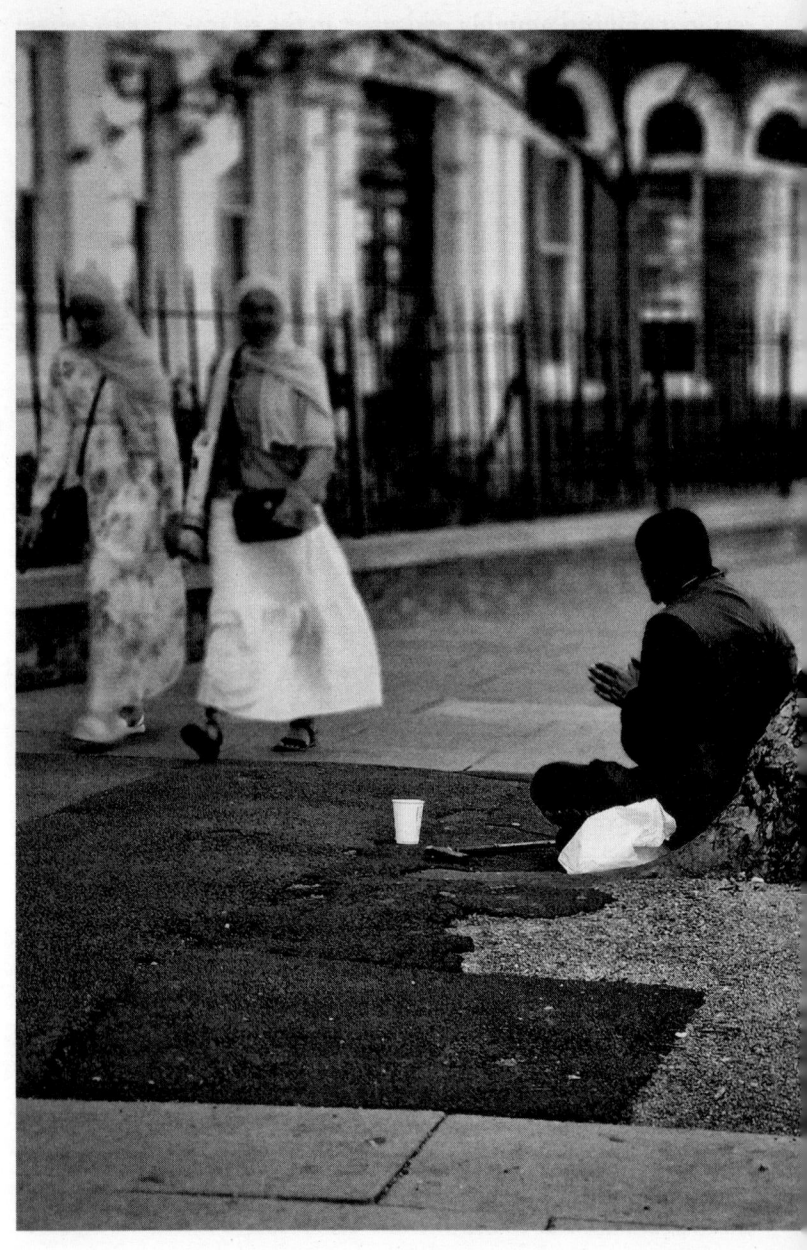

resilient and often highly educated, mature beyond their years. They are comfortable navigating both complex cultural and clinical contexts. I have met girls like Hanad's sister before, and I will meet many more. But each time I am impressed all over again.

I learn that for some time the family has been talking about Hanad spending some time back in either Kenya or the Netherlands, a chance to get away from the intensity of London. Hanad's presentation to A & E has confirmed the decision for the family, and it's Kenya that feels like the right change of environment. But I wonder if Hanad can survive all this change. If he hasn't been able to keep away from the dangers that thrive on London's streets, how will he manage in Kenya, where life is so much harder for his family there?

I know that Hanad and his family are bewildered by all the questions, and to some extent they are looking to health professionals like me and Kat to provide solutions, to tell them what to do. Is it better and safer for Hanad to stay in a city that has failed him, or should he go to Kenya, to a country he knows so little about? Should Hanad listen to his mother and sister? Or should he listen to his brothers on the streets, who have been encouraging him to stay in the city and fight, because that is what they do? I hope he will also listen to his heart, which is telling him that taking his own life isn't a solution, that there is hope – whether here or there – beyond the pain he's currently feeling.

I don't have all the answers. My role is to provide an assessment of Hanad's mental health, to evaluate his safety and work out whether he has plans to end his life or not, and to put forward a programme in which we can support him to feel safe. But what safety looks like for young people who are exposed to gang culture is open to debate. They often feel unsafe around their peers as well as around the police, and will do whatever is necessary to form structures to keep themselves safe. Sometimes, these very same structures – joining forces with a group of people who seem to be like them, for example – will turn against them. Violence among gang members and young people who grow up with each other is rife, and young people are often exploited by the people they know, their so-called 'friends' from school, college, or perhaps prison.

For Hanad and other vulnerable people like him who are confronted with these complex realities, there are few services available that can deal meaningfully with their needs. I think through the follow-up options.

I'd like Hanad to see his GP again, as he has had brief contact with his GP before, but I know the context has changed. His mental health has declined beyond stress, and he is showing signs of depression and is unsure of his safety. The system works for those who are obedient and consistent, for those who make, confirm and attend appointments. It is not designed with Hanad in mind, for those with more chaotic lives, who don't feel part of the mainstream, who are disengaged from society. His presentation in A & E meets criteria for a referral to a community mental-health team, who are well placed to work with patients like Hanad. This multi-disciplinary team of psychiatrists, psychologists, nurses, occupational therapists, psychotherapists, art therapists and support workers are able to offer a wide range of treatment options, including talking therapies. This system works well for those who choose to engage. But I know the system too well. Hanad's referral will float around for a while, long enough for most of the doctors, psychologists and nurses not to be able to see beyond his risk of violence. Even if he is offered an appointment, Hanad will struggle to make it because the clinic may be in a postcode that's dangerous for him to pass through, or the appointment will be in the morning, a time he'll struggle with because of his erratic sleep patterns. His case will eventually be closed because the service and the patient could not meet each other halfway.

I also consider the home treatment team (HTT), an excellent NHS service that provides treatment in the comfort of a patient's own home, or with some flexibility of meeting them wherever works best. Hanad would be a good candidate, but I am concerned that the HTT will not be able to visit him at home due to risks associated with gangs, and they might not be able to agree an alternative venue because of the postcode or street boundaries that Hanad has had to impose on himself to stay safe.

It's why it takes a service like the Gangs Unit to access a young person like Hanad. But the Gangs Unit is not widespread and doesn't cover the whole of London, let alone the whole of the country. It's another reason why some young people – too many young people – fall through the so-called safety net. The gaps are too wide. Hanad is in danger of becoming one of the ones we leave behind.

In the end, I decide that going to Kenya might just give Hanad a fresh chance – to grieve and to heal and to make sense of what he wants from his life.

I can only hope that he makes it there.

9. Zane: The House

> *'Private school children are being groomed by drug gangs as they are "less likely to be identified" by the police.'*

IT'S THE SUMMER OF 2018, the end of June. The picnics and sunglasses, sandals and summer dresses are out, despite the typically unreliable weather. England has recently made it to the semi-finals of the football World Cup; the agony and suspense that can hold an entire nation in thrall is upon us again. But when the lads lose out in the most dramatic fashion, the discussion around racism in football hits the headlines – and then it's gone again, simmering away in the background until next time. Another grand royal wedding is looming and the global media has outdone itself analysing the controversy of a new diversity within the British royal family.

For the rest of us, the summer carries on.

I am at home in north-east London, getting ready to leave for work, faffing with the contents of my rucksack, the radio burbling in the background. Issues of race and discrimination are increasingly popping up in the news, fuelled by the voice of the far right, which, worryingly, is gaining pace in Britain and across Europe. Even London, a city that prides itself on its multiculturism, is not free from it. My awareness of the problem is heightened because both my clients and my colleagues are highly sensitive to racism and injustice. Too often rightfully so. The National Health Service, a healthcare system that should be inclusive and representative of the diverse population it serves, isn't free from racism and discrimination. The experiences of minority nurses, midwives and doctors working on the frontline are harrowing – this, despite the expertise and innovation they bring into our healthcare system.

This morning, I pause and allow myself a moment before diving head first into busy London. Living and working in a big city can take its toll, particularly for mental-health professionals. The number of suicides is high and the rate of burnout among healthcare workers is increasing; I need to look after myself. I take steps to safeguard myself through daily rituals of yoga and meditation, and the occasional escape from the city. I've just enjoyed a long weekend of walks in Devon, which has worked wonders for my well-being, allowing me to reconnect with nature. But returning to the frontline after a break requires a moment of adjustment. This job is a calling. There is always another young person out there living in fear of violence, another family grappling with the trauma of knife crime. Today, I am heading out west, to Richmond, to meet a family I have been working with who, to their surprise, have been affected by youth violence and exploitation.

Zane is fifteen and attends a private weekly boarding school in Surrey. Over the weekend, he was stopped and searched by police while in the company of his new 'friend', a fifteen-year-old girl called Livi. The incident happened late in the evening, near St John's Wood Tube station. When police searched the pair, it was Zane who was found with the bag of cannabis. No drugs were found on Livi, and she failed to own up to any association with Zane – what he had thought of as a friendship. She was

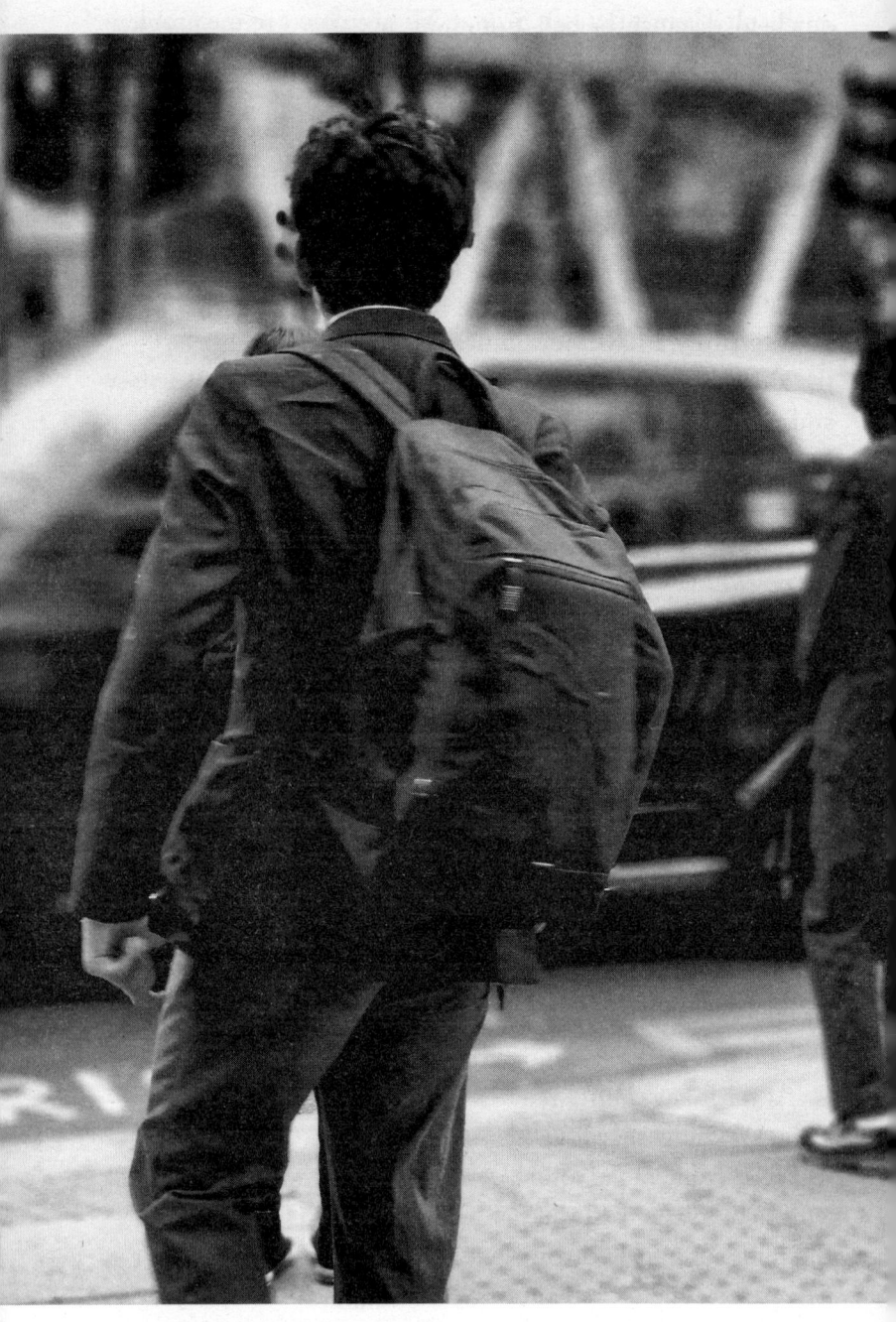

quick to distance herself from him and the cannabis in his pocket – cannabis she had supplied. Now, Zane is in trouble, both at home and out there on the streets.

He has been involved in a street fight – or was jumped, as young people call it – as he was walking alone along the canal between St John's Wood and Regent's Park. The brief attack, lasting less than fifteen seconds, was filmed and posted on social media to humiliate him, and to affirm the gang's power within their territory. I have viewed the disturbing video. The faces of the kids who attacked Zane are all partially covered by hoodies, and they're shouting, 'Posh boy!' Zane covers his head with his hands to defend himself and manages to stagger along the graffitied walls of the canal before finding his way out to the main road. Shocked onlookers appear horrified at the violence they're witnessing.

The attackers seem slightly younger than Zane, which to me and the Gangs Unit suggests that it was a strategy set up by older gang members to initiate the youngers into the gang. Zane's new iPhone was stolen in the process, and he was emotionally as well as physically bruised. It was soon after that attack that various team members spotted Zane hanging around with Livi, and concerns grew. Uncertain of his own world, Zane has found company – and what he has mistaken for security – on the streets. In view of the fight, the associations with young people known to be involved with criminality and exploitation, and the cannabis caution, Zane has been referred to the Gangs Unit, as he is deemed vulnerable.

At the Gangs Unit, we know that Zane is easy pickings for a gang. We know that Livi, his new friend, is often casually used to access vulnerable young people and draw them into local gang activity. As if all this wasn't enough, Zane's parents are in the midst of a toxic divorce and his father has already found a new partner and moved her into his new home. There's a tension in the family which is making it difficult for Zane and his twin sister Zara to thrive. His case was referred to me because of the emotional instability Zane is experiencing as a result of the divorce. And, since Zane comes from money, some of which has already been thrown at his well-being, there are complexities in coordinating his care, which falls between private and public mental-health services.

Zane's dad, Liam, is from Liverpool, born to Irish immigrants who migrated to England in the early sixties. Zane's mother, Priya, was born to Ugandan-Indian parents who fled Uganda to the United Kingdom after the country's expulsion of Asians in the early seventies. Liam and Priya, it seems, bonded over both being raised by immigrant parents who experienced adversity but established themselves in British society nonetheless. Like many immigrants who move to the UK, Zane's grandparents worked hard to provide for their children and, for Priya's Ugandan-Indian parents, a good education was paramount. Priya was educated at a boarding school in the south-west, and she and Liam wanted the same standard of education for their children.

Zane, like his mother, is academically able – good at maths and science, and, it's still hoped, heading towards a career in law or medicine. But it's that very academic strength, along with his mixed cultural heritage, that has led to Zane being bullied at school. When the bullying escalated, Zane sought out friendships that he believed would protect him from the bullying, but which turned out to be toxic. Zane, and to some extend Zara too, feels trapped between school and home. Both parents, his mother particularly, are angry that Zane's attention has been diverted away from his – or, more accurately, their – academic values. Liam, who leans conservative, is more shocked than anything else. He works as an executive for a development charity and he travels often. He's struggling to engage with the problem, and his response has been muted, inadequate, which has frustrated Priya further.

Since the police caution, Zane has gone to stay at his dad's house in Richmond to put some distance between him and the seething tensions at his mother's home in St John's Wood. Priya has sent me text messages filled with anxiety and concern for Zane, as any parent would. Yes, she is naturally worried that Zane has derailed his education and his future, but she seems equally annoyed that she has had to take time out of her work schedule as a university lecturer to support him with the troubles he – in her words – has 'brought upon himself'.

With Liam frozen in shock, Priya feels very alone in all this. She has been reluctant to reach out to her extended family for help because of the stigma attached to antisocial behaviour in their community. Worse, she knows they will probably blame all this on her because of the break-up of her marriage. In my work with young people exposed to gangs, I have looked after a wide range of young people from various demographics. Few of the families I have worked with have come from an elevated social class. Equally, Asian communities, of either Indian or Chinese heritage, also feature less in gang activities in London. The evidence base for why children of Indian or Chinese heritage appear to be protected from gang involvement and school exclusion is still very poor and is therefore largely anecdotal. Conversations I have had with community members suggest that it is probably due to these children being more likely to come from two-parent homes, units which are further strengthened by community cohesion. Class, too, is something of a protective factor, because with money you have so many more options to explore, including family activities that are not easily available to poorer families. Zane's family history is still somewhat vague to me, and at the moment I only have Priya's narrative to go on, but I'm eager to know more.

It is clear, however, that for Liam and Priya, in their mixed marriage and in the very busy modern lives they're leading, there seems to be less connection to their extended Indian-Asian family than is typical. This isolation is consistent with Western culture, and works for and against families. Creating distance allows people to live life on their own terms. But life can be harder when there's no support around you, particularly when you're raising a young family.

Priya has been clear with me: she loves her son deeply and wants him to come home to north-west London. But she's feeling overwhelmed at the moment. I can hardly blame her for not knowing what to do; she has no point of reference, as nothing like this has ever happened to her – or, indeed, to anyone she knows. These are issues she has only heard about, or read about – bad things which happen on the fringes of her neighbourhood. Not in her wildest dreams – or nightmares – did she ever imagine that gang activity would affect her family directly. And the impact is significant. Before Zane's cannabis incident and the fight by the canal, the twins had been spending two weeks together at one parent's house, followed by two weeks at the other. But now the even greater fallout between the parents has created a rift between the twins. Zane has chosen to spend more time with his dad, while Zara stays with her mum.

Zara is also academically bright, and she too has problems. She has been refusing food, either hiding it or purging. Her weight had dropped significantly enough for the school to notify the parents and suggest referring her to the local eating-disorder clinic. The parents, however, have opted to send Zara to a private specialist, as the pathway is much quicker. Both parents have had to acknowledge that the divorce may be having a negative effect on the twins. Priya's focus, she tells me, is on supporting Zara with an emerging eating disorder, and on keeping her job as an academic.

*

Children who attend private schools and have mental-health needs, which can and should be met by the local mental-health services, very easily fall between the cracks. When there are too many options on the table, it's easy for none to come through, as everyone assumes someone else is taking care of things. Also, compared to inner-city state schools, where safeguarding is everyday business, private schools do not always have sufficiently strong policies in place. In the private sector, where parents are paying hefty sums, a school may feel less empowered to challenge the very customers that keep their 'business' afloat. This can be further complicated by the fact that boarders within the private-education system will invariably be from different parts of the country, and sometimes from another country entirely, which makes the liaison needed to keep them safe at home and at school more difficult.

Things become even more complicated if parents have the resources to access private services, such as psychologists, psychiatrists or therapists, as the responsibilities of care become diluted, less joined up, and children are more likely to be forgotten. It's often the private providers who see the client first, because of their capacity to self-fund, but this does not necessarily guarantee a sustainable quality of care. Too often, some families can run out of money to fund the private care and then have to revert to NHS services. It can be messy.

Zane's parents have access to financial resources which they think can help Zane, but they are not emotionally competent enough to attend with conviction to the needs of either of their children. Liam has mentioned on the phone that the school picked up on Zane's change of behaviour; over the past few weeks, he has become irritable and his friendship groups at school have changed. But the school thought this could all be explained away by teenage hormones. Certainly, it appears that the school had wind of the parents' separation. And while Liam has acknowledged that the divorce proceedings may be having an adverse impact on the twins, neither he nor Priya ever imagined that the instability might predispose their son to gangs. It's a turn of events that's almost unfathomable in their otherwise polite lives. In their world, issues with gangs happen to other children, more likely from less privileged socio-economic backgrounds.

Had everyone been more vigilant, they might have identified these behavioural changes as red flags for gang involvement and exploitation. Other signs include a change of attitude towards girls, delinquency, impulsive and aggressive behaviours, social isolation and a fixation with social media. Individually, none of these signs suggests gang involvement. But when they are stacked up, they can indicate that a child is at risk. It's a crucial checklist.

Within a week of moving from referral to case management, I've gathered all the significant information on the family, including any clinical history relevant to my nursing interventions. It's now time to visit Zane at home – and I've decided it's best to see him at his dad's house in Richmond, as that's where he feels most comfortable. I'm hoping that our team interventions, supported by my nursing work, can turn things around not only for Zane, but for his whole family.

*

On the train to Richmond, ahead of the meeting with Liam and Zane, I try to get clear in my head exactly what has happened here. A fifteen-year-old boy from an affluent family is struggling with his emotions, and the system which should have supported him hasn't performed. Left to his own devices, Zane looked to cannabis to cope with the stress in his life – the bullying at school and his parents' divorce. His supplier was using a girl from a local estate, someone who pretended to be Zane's friend, to get the drugs to him; essentially, Livi was acting as the gang's runner. Tasked with befriending Zane, perhaps even flirting with him, her job was to draw him further into the gang.

And Zane had fallen for it.

In Livi, he had found a smoking partner, someone streetwise, worldly, and far more exciting than the biddable children he'd grown up with. She quickly became someone he could confide in about his feelings. Though divided by class, they were bound by two commonalities: Livi too comes from a broken home, and Livi too is of mixed heritage. She lives with her white mother and is estranged from her Black father. Zane had briefly mentioned Livi to his dad, but Liam hadn't paid much attention. Teenagers' lives revolve around friendships, he'd thought. It was good that Zane was expanding his network.

Liam was attentive enough to know that Zane was occasionally smoking cannabis, and this alarmed him. Trying to put aside the acrimonious dynamics of the divorce, he reached out to Priya to ensure that she too addressed the cannabis issue with Zane when he stayed with her. But the toxicity between them overshadowed their attempts to parent consistently. The message they were giving Zane became disjointed and inconsistent.

Change can affect even well-functioning adults negatively. Children, however, often experience change particularly powerfully, and the associated risks run across all demographics. Children will sense tension between parents or guardians, a tension that the children then soak up. And they are an easy punchbag – metaphorically and sometimes literally – for irritable and angry adults. Tensions in a relationship can play out as full-blown domestic violence, emotional or financial abuse. An assumption

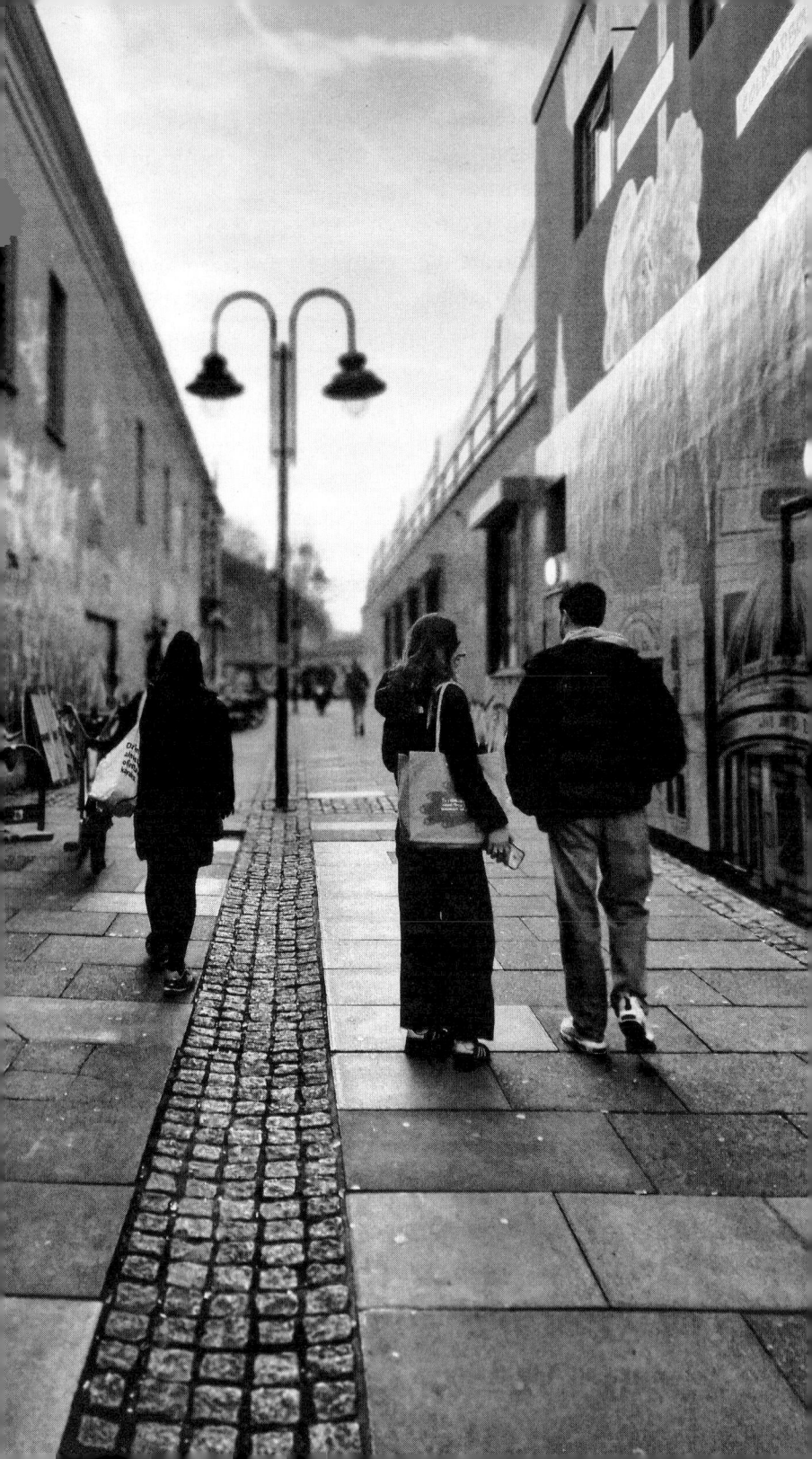

is often made that middle-class women like Priya are not exposed to domestic violence because they have the resources to explore other options, to extricate themselves from an ugly situation, but this is far from the truth. On the contrary, there is evidence to suggest that women who are breadwinners are highly exposed to domestic violence, particularly in cultures that place a lot of value on patriarchy and masculinity.

While there is nothing to suggest that domestic violence has been an issue between Liam and Priya, I have to keep it in mind as a possibility.

Some children can't express their sense of grief and loss at the collapse of a marriage and, with it, their family life. They aren't able to navigate the uncertainties of when they will see their parents again and the emotional turmoil that comes with supervised contacts or brief visits, which are often marked by materialism to make up for the absence of daily parenting. These issues can increase feelings of anxiety and depression in young people.

Where parents leave a relationship and quickly move on to a new one, often neglecting their children's emotional needs in pursuit of their own, some children will struggle to adjust to new partners, new schools, step-siblings or new homes. Adolescents who are transitioning through these changes can be particularly vulnerable. All this can affect their school performance, their ability to trust, their sense of security, and may trigger changes in their eating habits. A good school will be proactive in supporting children going through these social and cultural changes.

Some young people find solace in using drugs as a coping mechanism. What starts off as mild cannabis use can escalate to harder drugs, such as crystal meth, cocaine and sometimes even heroin. Of course, some children might use all of these drugs and not come into contact with gangs – if the drugs arrive via friends, for example, rather than being purchased directly. However, their use increases the chances of a meeting happening.

The loss of a parent through the breakdown of a relationship can play out in many ways. Some children feel guilty about their parents separating, and this might lead to self-harming, intense suicidal ideation, poor self-worth and hopelessness. Children do best when parents talk to them about how the separation is affecting them, and give credence to their emotions. It's OK to feel anxious. It's OK to feel that the rug has been pulled away from under your feet. It's OK to worry about how this new-look family is going to work.

Liam and Priya had grown apart in their marriage, each finding solace in their work. They're now blaming each other for the cracks that have formed within their family. Liam and Priya are mid-battle; Zane and Zara are the casualties.

*

The sunshine is bright as I emerge out of Richmond Underground station. It's a wealthy area, with inviting shops all along the high street. Vegan muffins and fresh Scandinavian sandwiches are displayed in a cafe's gleaming windows. The aroma of coffee drifts through the air. Well-heeled locals are walking their equally well-heeled dogs.

It's a short walk from the station to Zane's home. Passing through a wrought-iron gate and up a short garden path, I knock on a wooden door that has been painted a vivid, glossy orange. There is a bark in response. I can hear Liam trying to shoo the dog away, but when, after a pause, he opens the door, one hand is holding the collar of a small dog to stop it leaping up at me.

'She's fine, really. Her bark is worse than her bite,' he says by way of a greeting.

I look down at a cute brown-and-white Jack Russell terrier with rather beautiful eyes.

'Come on, Polly, calm down, calm down. There's a good girl,' Liam assures her.

I slip my shoes off in a hallway that's filled with large pictures of nature: mountains, glaciers and rivers in countries I cannot instantly name. The Afghan runner that leads away from the front door is dominated by a deep red that ties into the hues of an armchair in the living room. With one eye on the boisterous Polly, I take in the well-stocked bookshelf, which also showcases photos of Zane and Zara, from newborn babies to teenagers. One of the photos is signed: *Dear Zane and Zara, love always, Grandad.*

I move closer, curious to know more about Zane's home life.

Liam is of average build and perhaps in his early forties. His hair is wavey and short, his accent crisp and brusque. His conduct is purposeful, collected. He has mannerisms which suggest compassion – he does, after all, work in the charity sector – but also power. Yet I can sense his powerlessness in the situation that brings us together today. Zane's new-found associations have brought the world of gangs into Liam's comfortable life, a life he has worked hard for, and his anxiety feels urgent.

'Are you alright, darling?' a woman's raised voice reaches us from down the hallway. Liam's new partner.

Liam acknowledges her, but is focused on settling the dog. Polly is taking up time he doesn't really have. I sense that he wants to get to the crux of things as quickly as possible, and that his time today, and every day, is pressured. He has many questions that need answering – the who, the what and the why of it all. I watch him fuss around with the dog for a moment, then I move forward and pet Polly on her head and across her lean shoulders. It's a friendly gesture from the stranger on her turf, and it calms her down.

As the dog settles, Liam turns his attention to me. 'Zane is upstairs in his room,' he says. 'Since this whole thing happened with the police, he hardly leaves his room.'

I'm not surprised by this.

'You've got to help me understand this,' Liam says, as we sit down. 'How on earth could Zane be found with so much cannabis on him? I knew he was smoking a joint here and there, but to be caught with such an amount . . .' He trails off, and I wait for him to continue. 'Did someone set him up?' he asks. 'They must have done. Zane is such an easy target.'

Liam's hypothesis may well be right. It's highly likely that Livi moved fast and passed the cannabis on to Zane as the police closed in on them, ridding herself of all blame and any criminal outcome. It's a move she will have mastered from the 'elders', a move that has left Zane exposed.

For a moment, we sit quietly. Sunlight streams through the slatted wooden blinds. A clutch of Lycra-clad runners flash by the large bay window. But the air in the room is heavy with tension. The dog gets up and pads softly out of the room. It's a beautiful home, but misery lives here too. Even so, I have to wonder how a child from a background like this gets lured into gangs.

'Dorcas, help me understand this,' Liam pleads. 'My world is so far removed from this stuff. I spend my time standing up for people around the world who have no access to food, water or education. But I know absolutely nothing about these London gangs.'

In some ways, Liam is right to be bewildered. The London Borough of Richmond is not high on gang prevalence, certainly not compared to other boroughs, such as Brent, Lambeth, Westminster and Enfield. We know from academic research that there's a link between class and gangs, and that, if you are Black and from a lower class, you are more likely to be arrested or searched by the police purely on spec. Zane's association with

Livi – mixed race and working class – increased his risk of stop, search and arrest. Had Zane been smoking cannabis alone in Richmond, he may not have been stopped in the first place. This leniency probably wouldn't have been afforded to a young Black boy living on a council estate.

We live in an unjust world, and Zane has been lucky. He was stopped and searched in an affluent area of London and was cautioned; we have to acknowledge that the result might have been different for a young person of Black ethnicity stopped in a deprived area. These deeply contested issues can put a strain on the relationship between the police and the communities they serve. But I am proud to have worked with a great number of compassionate and caring officers who see the bigger picture and try to do their bit to close some of these societal gaps.

Just as crossing postcodes can be dangerous for gang members, crossing the class lines has made Zane's social environment more hazardous. None of this jeopardy had previously registered with Liam.

The front door slams: Liam's partner has taken the dog out for a walk, perhaps to give us space. I don't know what part she's playing in all of this, if any. The introduction of a new partner will have been felt by Zane, though. Liam offers tea and I oblige him, if only to buy time to help him calm down. If he's calm, we'll be able to have a more meaningful conversation.

With his trembling hands now gripped around a cup of tea, he leans towards me. He tells me that Zane has been receiving messages from Livi saying that he owes £2,000 for the cannabis that was taken by the police and that he needs to pay it back as soon as possible. Livi doesn't say much more than this, but the tone is increasingly threatening – so much so that Zane felt the need to share what's happening with his father. He's scared. He wants Liam to pay out the £2,000 and make the matter go away. Liam and Priya have discussed this, and are conflicted. Liam, being the more emotional and nervous of the two, is of the opinion that they should report the texts to the police. Priya is more cautious, worried that involving the police might create more problems for Zane. It's a landscape they know little about. How to navigate it is difficult. It's this lack of understanding that the gangs are leaning in to; they see the family's vulnerability as a lucrative market they're keen to tap.

Liam and I spend some time talking through the issues. I'm ready to make full use of this teachable moment.

I carefully tell him about how gangs work and how good they are at exploiting vulnerable young people. Liam can't understand how Zane's new 'friend', Livi, might have been part of the stitch; his own life has been sheltered from these particular social issues. I am compassionate as I explain how the gangs' networks operate; I don't wish to suggest that he, as a parent, should have been more observant. As I speak, it feels like a new idea is taking shape: a much-needed educational programme designed for well-to-do families who only hear about gangs from a distance, never imagining that their own children could be affected.

Moments later, I hear a fuss in the hallway and the front door slams again. This time, I realize, it can only be Zane storming out of the house. I stand up quickly and, through the window, am just in time to watch him disappear into the streets, his hood pulled up over his head. His strides are purposeful. He cannot get away fast enough – from me? Liam stands up too and watches his son disappear into what feels like a wilderness.

I wonder what's going through Zane's mind. There are a number of emotions that could be at play. He is probably embarrassed because he allowed a girl to 'play' him. He will still be bruised, at least metaphorically, from the canal fight that was shared widely on social media. And he may be feeling guilty because of the disruption he has brought into his parents' lives when they're already grappling with work-related stress and the fallout from the divorce, as well as Zara's struggle with an eating disorder.

'I'm worried about Zane,' Liam says, still gazing out of the window. 'This is all too much for him.'

There is good reason to worry.

'Dorcas,' he continues, 'two thousand pounds is nothing out of my pocket. Do you think I should just pay it, and relieve Zane of the stress? Should we just report Livi to the police?'

Liam's anxiety is clouding his judgement. While I appreciate the urgency he feels in wanting to help his son, I fear he's at risk of making a bad situation worse. It may be true that £2,000 is a drop in the ocean for him, but the gangs realize that too and are looking to draw from that potentially bottomless well; by giving them money now, Liam will be confirming that they have hit the jackpot. Their demands thereafter will be relentless. And Zane is not the only child at risk. Liam may think paying the money will also release Livi from her obligations to the gang, but that is not within his control. And it's certainly not something I can help with.

My work as a mental-health nurse is to implement the psychological tools which enable young people to heal. When it comes to gangs and money, I'm not the expert. But the youth workers in our team know how money moves within gangs, how it's managed and the structures that gangs create to balance income and outgoings; they will be better able to navigate this area with Liam. I reassure him that, in the next day or so, one of our experienced youth workers will get in touch. Kofi is best placed to advise on the money that's involved here. He understands the depth of the pit that Zane has fallen into and, most importantly, how to support him while he tries to get out of it.

I need to be clear with Liam about my remit. If I can help

to manage my clients' anxieties, a thinking space will open up to enable Zane and his dad to deal with their situation with clear heads. All I can do is tell Liam that he is probably trying to apply his corporate problem-solving skills to a situation he knows little about, and I advise him that sometimes it's more beneficial to step back and take advice from those best positioned to offer it. He nods wearily.

'Let's get some more tea,' he suggests.

It's the solution to any problem, at least for a moment.

Liam leads me into the generous kitchen at the back of the house. A marble-topped island sits in the middle of the room and an Aga is set against the wall. Double doors open out onto a manicured lawn, upon which a large Buddha statue sits. I take in my surroundings and marvel again at the contrast between this and the council flats, and indeed prison visiting areas, in which I see my other clients.

I hear some soft footsteps behind us and swing around.

'Please meet my girlfriend, Beverly,' Liam says.

Beverly strolls across the kitchen to Liam and leans into his brief embrace.

'Lovely to meet you,' she says to me. I detect the lingering traces of a Yorkshire accent. 'Isn't it terrible, what's going on out there. It's awful.'

There's something about her breezy tone that suggests Zane is far down her list of priorities. Still, she is here.

Over our second cup of tea, I confirm that Kofi will give Liam all the guidance he needs on what to do next regarding the money. From my perspective, I suggest that he keeps a close and caring eye on Zane, and we talk about the mental-health issues that adolescents who are in this predicament can experience. I have to tell him that they can pose a risk to themselves through self-harm or suicide, and I register his shock when I say this. Zane is lucky to be among his family, I tell Liam, but he's alone nevertheless, with no real outlet for his emotions, particularly if he doesn't want to talk to me.

There's rarely just one reason for someone to take their own life. It's always an accumulation of factors, and the use of drugs and alcohol can increase the risk. Suicide cuts across demographics. In the Global North, death by suicide is particularly high among young white males. And, in rural environments, it's particularly high among farmers – somewhat ironically, the very community that Liam supports through his development work.

When adolescents are struggling, they are more likely to confide in their friends than their family. If Zane has expressed any thought of suicide, it may well have been to Livi. But now Livi is out of the picture and the feeling that he can't trust his so-called friends makes Zane even more vulnerable.

*

As I am putting my shoes back on and preparing to leave, Zane returns home. He bursts through the front door and slams it shut behind him with a force that makes us all jump. His face is still very deliberately half covered by his hoodie and he avoids any eye contact with us, looking down at the floor. A tense silence immediately descends and I quickly jump in to offer Zane empathy. While his father is fumbling for the right words, Zane needs to hear something, to know that he is not alone.

'You alright, Zane?' I ask pleasantly. It's a simple acknowledgement of his presence. 'I'm off now, but can we catch up some other time?'

For the sake of his ego and need to feel in control, I don't expect him to speak to me while his parents are around. I'm allowing Zane to take charge.

'When can we catch up, Zane? It's really important that we do.' I move a little closer to him, in search of eye contact.

I'm offering trust. 'Can we catch up when you're next at your mum's?' I persist, and it pays off.

'Yeah, sure,' he eventually replies, stepping around us and beginning to walk up the stairs. Polly the dog follows him with her eyes.

'See you later, Zane,' I call after him.

I want him to know that he's important. That I care. That my presence in his home is an act of compassion. That he is valued and his safety is high on my agenda. He glances back at me as he climbs the stairs, too well brought up to ignore me completely, and our eyes lock for a moment. He sees me – and perhaps realizes that I'm here to offer hope. I need him to hang in there, because I believe there is always hope.

I watch Liam gaze at his son as he disappears upstairs, lost in his own thoughts.

'Shall I walk you out?' he asks. Without waiting for an answer, he follows me into the front garden and quietly closes the orange door behind us, leaving Polly barking away and Beverly holding onto her tightly.

Liam is yearning for a psychological safe space in which to be honest about his feelings. And I allow him that.

'Look, this is a hard journey, very hard,' he says to me as we walk past the neighbouring homes with their sash windows flung open to the summer breeze. 'I don't know how to do this. How can I be a better dad for Zane? I know how to provide for him, practically, but I am not used to this emotional stuff.'

I let him get it all out.

'My daughter's also struggling . . . I want to be there for both of them.'

We pause by the corner shop, in front of newspaper front pages splashed with pictures of the royal family, a story which has pushed the racism in football debate off the agenda.

When I turn and look into Liam's eyes, I see fear and

hopelessness. He is almost defeated by this. Parents whose children are affected by gang culture often suffer in silence. There are rarely psychologically safe outlets in which they can express themselves. Some parents are stigmatized by their own communities, blamed for their children's delinquent and disorderly behaviours. Although Liam has Beverly by his side, I suspect that he's carrying this mental-health burden alone.

'You're doing well, under the circumstances,' I reassure him.

As we continue on to the Tube station, I share some of the psycho-education advice that we use in clinics for adults struggling with low-level mental-health distress. We talk about the need to ensure he is emotionally available to Zane, the importance of listening to Zane – both his verbal and non-verbal communication. And I explain that, above all, it's essential that he validates Zane's feelings. We discuss the power of silence and how to read silence and work with it. Adolescents will often disappear into their shell and isolate themselves – just as Zane has been going to his room. This isolation increases the risk of self-harm and depression. It is precisely at this difficult time that they need someone to talk to.

Liam admits to me that his own upbringing was very different, that he grew up in a large Irish family where emotions were not expressed. His parents rarely told him that they loved him; he simply had to assume that they did. Now, he's having to learn a new, emotionally expressive language. And he'll commit to this work because he loves his children.

*

In our next group meeting, I bring the case forward for discussion. It's in some ways ordinary, in the sense that we are used to dealing with the interconnected complexities of health, social and cultural challenges. However, most of the young people we work with are casualties of structural inequalities – school exclusion, domestic violence, racism and discrimination, poor community cohesion and living in an environment that is highly exposed to criminality. But Zane ticks only one of these boxes; on the contrary, for the most part, he has been experiencing life at the other end of the privilege spectrum, in a somewhat rarefied atmosphere.

The group asks questions about the family that get me thinking even more deeply.

'Why, over the years, has Liam placed greater importance on his work than on his son?'

'The parents are probably used to throwing money at every problem, that's why they're struggling to comprehend the complexity of gang culture.'

'Is Zara's eating disorder her way of coping with a difficult family situation?'

'If Zane continues to use cannabis, he could be excluded from the private school, and that would cause him more problems, at least mentally.'

'What's Zane's mum like? I wonder if she's more empathetic than the dad?'

Then our group therapist makes an enlightened suggestion.

'Shouldn't we be viewing this through a post-traumatic stress disorder framework?' she asks. 'What Zane has been through is nothing short of traumatic.'

There is a general acknowledgement that there's still quite a lot we don't fully know about the family. But we do know that Zane is being exploited. The PTSD framing presents an opportunity to design my nursing interventions very specifically with that in mind.

Fired up, the group suggests more ideas.

'If Kofi is working with Liam and Zane, perhaps you can both try to work with the mum, too.'

'There's still some trauma work to be done. It's about identifying the right parent to work with as an ally.'

'Yes, suicide or self-harm is a risk, but the sooner Zane gets help, the better his outcomes might be.'

'We're lucky that the summer break is about to start, which gives a good window of opportunity to do some meaningful work with him before he goes back to boarding school.'

I take it all in.

My first action point is to text Zane, who agrees to meet with me at his mum's house. For Zane, the geographical area in which his exploitation took place may be triggering – and perhaps that's why he has recently chosen to spend most of his time out in Richmond. However, by agreeing to meet me in St John's Wood, it suggests that he's ready to immerse himself in the therapeutic work that's required to get him through this trauma.

I also ask Priya if I can meet with her, separately. She'll be able to help me fully understand and support Zane.

*

Around midday on a Thursday afternoon, I take the bus from Oxford Circus to St John's Wood. It's an area of obvious affluence, peppered with some council-estate housing. If poverty is a fact of life, then I prefer a mixed neighbourhood, where there's greater social integration. Polarization fuels division and makes inequality much harder to tackle, as there's so little investment in a place where only poorer people live. Here, where wealth on one street meets poverty on the next, it's easy to see how Zane and Livi's worlds collided.

I have been thinking through the PTSD work that I need to do with Zane. Some healthcare professionals are of the view that PTSD is over-medicalized. Joel Paris, a Canadian psychiatrist, explores its over-diagnosis in his book *Myths of Trauma* and elsewhere, and makes the case that psychiatry has lost its way by trying to pathologize almost all of life's inevitable misfortunes. Some clinicians I've worked with are of the view that the over-diagnosis of PTSD means it's open to abuse and, more importantly, its prevalence takes focus away from those patients who are genuinely experiencing it. I would argue that the life events of the adolescents I'm working with – events such as stabbings, street fights, exploitation and even gun violence – do meet the criteria for PTSD, where symptoms typically include flashbacks, anxiety, poor sleep, aggression or developing poor coping mechanisms such as increased use of drugs or alcohol.

All of this is in my mind as I ring Priya's bell. A middle-aged British Asian woman of average build opens the door. Her long black hair is streaked with grey and is tied up with a beautiful bow on the top of her head. A few strands fall loose around her face. Like Liam, she has come to the door with a pet. She's holding a cat, which she strokes as she smiles and introduces herself. I reciprocate and offer her my nursing credentials. She welcomes me warmly into the house.

The hallway is lined with books, some clearly rather old, both hardcovers and paperbacks; they all look as though they've been well read. I scan the titles, distracted by the corridor library. Priya gives a little cough to get my attention, and I chuckle as I ease myself out of my own wonder and back into the real world.

'Zane's upstairs. He knows you're coming, so maybe you and I could have a chat first and you can catch up with him later?' she suggests.

While clearly vulnerable, Priya immediately strikes me as more in control than Liam, and I soon discover why. As a university lecturer, she has become well versed in gangs, exploitation and violence, as it occasionally presents itself in the university's grounds. The conversation is similar to those I've had with schoolteachers; the risk factors for their young people are pretty much the same. But, like Liam, what Priya hadn't expected was that her own son would find himself involved in gang activity.

Helpfully, she has some reflections to share.

She recalls meeting Livi, who came to the house looking for Zane. She was, Priya tells me, a likeable girl, well dressed, polite, with good eye contact. She seemed sweet, though a little nervous – perhaps about meeting her friend's mum, Priya had thought. Perhaps about supplying Zane with cannabis, she now realizes. Priya became worried when she noticed Zane was secretly smoking cannabis in his room on the top floor, the smell lingering in the air. Then he began to do it openly in the house when she wasn't there – always denying it, despite the aromatic evidence.

She confesses that, since the separation and now divorce, she has immersed herself in her work, all the more intensely when the twins are away at school.

'If only I'd paid more attention to what Livi was doing with Zane,' she says with regret in her voice. But then she changes tack, taking a more practical approach. 'But what can you do? You have to give teenagers space. You can't keep them strapped to your hip.' Finally, she arrives at the clinical statistics. 'You know, in any year, one in four of us is likely to experience poor mental health,' she tells me. 'And pretty much one in four children, too. Emotional disorders. Anxiety. Depression. Young women, sixteen to twenty-four, are particularly high risk – it's twice as high for them.'

She has done her homework, I'll give her that. And I can see that, for Priya, it's easier to focus on the broader picture, rather than the parenting issues that are specific to her situation. But no amount of statistical analysis will help Zane right now. She needs to focus on him, not the data.

'We have thrown a lot of money into trying to protect him,' she continues, with a sigh, 'and then this . . .'

I can see that there are similarities between Liam and Priya in the way they're reacting to the situation. Priya may have an understanding of what gang culture is – she's better informed, more measured and less prone to panic – but she is equally perplexed about what to do. They both want to be allies for Zane, but neither knows how to step up.

There's a movement behind me, and I turn to see Zane.

He goes straight to his mum and takes the cat from her, stroking it smoothly, almost therapeutic in his manner. His hood is down, and by allowing us to see his face it feels as though, this time, he has decided to be fully present. He knows that Priya and I have been talking about him and, as if to show me how mature he can be, he takes control of the conversation: 'I'm alright to have a chat with the nurse on my own, now, Mum.'

It's quite a transformation from the sullen door-slammer I last encountered. I wonder if, in the meantime, Zane has realized that the one person he can depend on is himself, that his two parents are not going to be much help to him this time. He wouldn't be the first young person I've worked with to figure that out. Priya leaves us alone in the kitchen.

*

I have a simple question to start things off: 'Are you alright, Zane?'

He opens up almost immediately.

It's the first time I'm hearing his version of events, and I don't take it lightly that Zane feels safe to share everything with me. He says he has been thinking a lot about the incident, from the first time he met Livi, to being arrested for carrying weed, to the threatening text messages he has received from her.

'It's crazy, though . . .'

Zane is lost in thought. He has a lot of processing to do. As his nurse, I'm here to unpack some of those thought processes with him.

After a while, he begins again: 'I've heard about people taking advantage of other people, but I never thought it would happen to me. She just came across like a nice person, someone I could talk to.'

I wait.

'With all this happening, I just thought she was someone I could talk to,' he says again.

I sit and listen to Zane, watching him closely. This is his therapeutic space, where he can speak his mind and free himself of his burden. He uses the space well. He seems to have Priya's critical-thinking skills and Liam's anxiety, but he is much more reflective than either of his parents and appears to want to learn from this experience. His discomfort lingers, but he has learned an invaluable lesson. He is still suffering, but his suffering is important.

'The whole thing still gets to me, though. I still wake up sometimes in a sweat and panic . . .'

Zane tells me that he has been doing some work with Kofi around managing the expectations and demands that have continued to come from Livi's associates. And I know Kofi is having conversations with Zane about readjusting to his life back in school and dealing with the rumours about his arrest and caution that might follow him there. Kofi will have warned Zane about some of his peers who might want to humiliate him further, feeding off the film of the fight, or those who might want to draw him deeper into criminality now that he has brushed up against the law. This is a juncture at which many young people arrive and, without the right sort of mentoring, they can take the wrong path.

I discuss some PTSD coping mechanisms with Zane. I tell him about mindfulness, the importance of taking regular exercise, and ways to divert his thoughts when he's feeling overwhelmed. Zane reminds me that he doesn't feel safe walking around some parts of St John's Wood due to the attack and the falling-out with Livi. I hear that, and I acknowledge this wholly; it will take time before he regains his confidence. I suggest that he takes advantage of the greenery in Richmond; the emphasis is on getting some fresh air to free the mind, in whatever shape or form that is possible. We discuss ways to manage his emotions, which include regulating his sleep, reducing impulsive behaviours, adopting a problem-solving approach and talking through decisions with those he trusts.

This journey of transitioning from unhealthy behaviours, such as smoking cannabis, into healthy behaviours, such as exercise and mindfulness, is hard work. It takes time and a complete change of mindset. It's difficult for adults and even more so for adolescents, especially in this digital age where rest is hard to come by, but I am confident Zane is already on the right track.

'You know what I want to do . . .' he says, thinking aloud. 'I want to show this whole experience through music. I want to write songs and make sense of it through making something.'

I smile in validation of his vision.

There is a strong relationship between the arts and mental health, a relationship which is too often unexplored in the treatment of young people who experience violence in the settings in which I work. Drawing, painting, and music in particular, can be a way for those living with mental illness to engage and express their feelings, to reduce stress and anxiety by lowering cortisol levels. It can help to improve mood. It's a non-medical approach that I'm all in favour of. That Zane is looking to the arts to help express his own trauma fills me with so much hope for his future.

Zane whips out his phone to shows me some lyrics, words

he is putting together for a song. His eyes brighten as he talks me through what he has in mind. And I think that perhaps everyone involved here will eventually be able to look back on this incident as a catalyst for change; greater things lie ahead for this young man.

'How is Zara doing?' I ask.

As twins, Zane's mental-health recovery is linked to Zara's.

He pauses for a moment, and a look of concern returns to his face. 'She's doing alright,' he eventually says, but without certainty. 'She has a therapist. Maybe she could do with doing some music as well . . .'

I don't want to pressure Zane to dwell on Zara's care, and I know that eating disorders in adolescents are complex and multi-faceted in their causes and treatment. He tells me that the NHS waiting lists are long – and I sadly acknowledge this fact, and that this delay in receiving attention prolongs the suffering. Fortunately for this family, Zara is accessing private healthcare. Liam and Priya are balancing a lot – a child affected by trauma through gang activity, the other with eating disorders and anxiety. It's a heavy burden, but they are focused, now, on what needs to be done.

Zane shouts to his mother that we're winding up, and Priya reappears so swiftly I wonder if she has been listening at the door. I smile at her.

'I'm pleased to say that Zane is taking something from this experience,' I tell her, and she nods and smiles in response.

There are seedlings of recovery here, and we're both keen to see them nurtured. With care, Zane is moving away from the dark roads of exploitation towards personal growth.

*

In the evening, I walk across Primrose Hill towards Camden Town, taking a moment to breathe in London's fresh air and enjoy the always impressive view. I think of Zane and reflect on the place of deep vulnerability he has come from, and his journey towards something positive. I want this for each and every young person who is exposed to or affected by the city's gangs, but, in order to achieve this, we need to do more to ensure that there are trained nurses to work with our young people, to help them navigate their complex mental-health needs. We are still leaving far too many behind, from all sorts of different backgrounds, with different stories to tell. And if young people in London are not safe, then none of us truly are. When our young people thrive, we all thrive.

10. Alex: The School

'Too many children, including some as young as eleven, are carrying knives because they feel unsafe and see this as a form of protection.'

THE SCHOOL'S WAITING-ROOM WALLS, covered from floor to ceiling with graffiti art that's stylish and bold, strike me as remarkable. Each piece sends the imagination soaring far away from a grey inner-London comprehensive school and all its challenges on a drab winter morning. But, in case I forget where I am, the sound of children is a constant reminder that this is a living, breathing space. Their noise is sometimes close by — a wall not of art, but of sound — and at other times is nothing more than a murmur somewhere in the background.

A few of them dawdle past the main office, where I'm sitting on a sofa that has seen better days. They're dressed scrappily in dark-blue uniforms with white — and not so white — shirts, shoving each other as schoolchildren tend to do. Whether it's in bonding or intimidation is unclear; the line is often blurred. They glance into the waiting room with no interest, almost looking through me as I continue waiting patiently for Renee, Alex's sister, to arrive.

Alex is one of my clients. He's on the verge of being excluded from school for fighting with another boy in class and then, just when that tussle was being resolved, bringing a knife into school. Alex has been referred to my clinic to manage his anger and poor emotional regulation, both of which stem, at least in part, from his autism. It's an element of his character that Renee understands and negotiates well. But the school is less sympathetic to his needs and more focused on what it calls his 'behavioural difficulties' and the problems they're creating for the staff. Rather than supporting Alex, the school is saying he cannot stay here.

Renee and I are meeting Ms Rodney, the headteacher, who is leading on the school exclusion programme. I am a little anxious, anticipating a difficult meeting. Renee feels Ms Rodney isn't interested in her brother, and I'm inclined to agree. How the school deals with Alex is important. He is treading turbulent waters. Renee and I are battling for solutions, trying to find a positive way forward for him, but we feel as though we're on our own.

That Renee cares deeply about Alex's well-being has been evident from the moment I received the referral. Miles, the youth worker on the case, made it clear that my main contact would be Renee. At just nineteen years old, she has a good grasp of how schools operate, having been through the same school herself so recently. She too faced some challenges here, though she has now found herself a good job in the retail sector.

Renee is bright, socially and culturally attuned. She and Alex are typical London kids, with a parental heritage that sits between two lineages: Polish on their mother's side and Caribbean on their father's. They are growing up in a multicultural London that presents them with both great opportunities and considerable challenges. Renee is determined to carve out a future for herself that upends the societal narrative for a young

Black girl growing up on a council estate and attending a poorly rated school.

Her innate resilience positions her well for navigating the system with more ease than her parents have managed. While both parents have been physically present for their children, they have proved less emotionally equipped to deal with life's challenges. As a consequence, home is filled with heightened emotions. Their mother is struggling with anxiety. Their father is calmer, but only because he chooses to smoke cannabis, regularly excusing himself from parental responsibilities, leaving Renee to fill in the gaps. It's a common enough story.

I flick through my phone and look for a message from Renee. Freshly arrived in my unread texts, I find one telling me she's running slightly late. She has struggled to get time off from work, finally securing permission to leave her busy marketing department only at the last minute.

It's a lot to ask of her and this isn't the first time I am having to meet her here. We were here just a couple of weeks ago, when Alex was involved in a fight. Having fallen for Chantel, a girl lower down the school, he had written her a poignant love letter on Snapchat, which she had promptly shared with some friends. From there, it had gone viral, finally landing in the hands – or on the screen – of a boy who claimed to be the girl's current boyfriend. Alex was widely mocked, humiliated and ridiculed. For a young person with autism trying to process new emotions, this public gallery proved too cruel. Embracing his vulnerability, his so-called school friends whipped up the gossip, setting the two boys against each other. It was Renee who had messaged me to say that Alex had been involved in a fight, asking if I could come to the school with her that afternoon to talk to the head.

In the fight's aftermath, a teaching assistant was assigned to meet with Alex to debrief and offer some low-level conflict resolution. Alex had innocently informed the teaching assistant

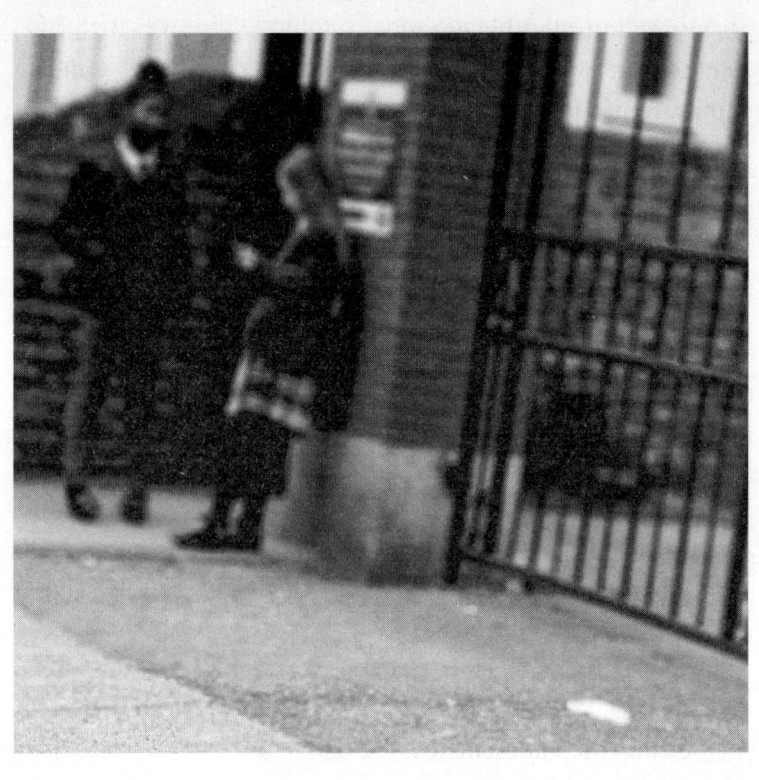

that he had a knife in his rucksack – brought to school because he felt the need to protect himself. The teaching assistant had escalated the case to the head, and now he is facing exclusion from mainstream education. The alternative – that Alex attend a Pupil Referral Unit – is too dire to contemplate. Alex has unwittingly turned his entire world upside down, with reverberations at every level, including within his already troubled family. Renee is devastated.

Ms Rodney arrives shortly after a flustered Renee, notified by the receptionist that her visitors are finally here. She's dressed in a severe grey suit that matches her steely manner. Her brunette hair is neatly tied back in a ponytail. She does not smile. She has come prepared for business.

Renee, I can see, is completely wound up, a coiled spring, and doesn't give Ms Rodney time to breathe before launching in. 'So, you're going to exclude my brother, just like that,' she blurts out. 'Do you know what those PRUs are like?'

Slightly taken aback, Ms Rodney draws a steady breath and, in a measured voice, explains: 'The school has a very clear policy on carrying knives. Very clear. We have a duty to keep all the children safe, including Alex.'

It's a statement of fact to which Renee finds it impossible to respond.

Seizing the moment, Ms Rodney quickly goes on: 'But, please, come with me to my office, where we can sit down and discuss it all fully.' She signals for me and Renee to follow her down a short corridor, and we silently oblige.

In the rather more subdued office, designed perhaps to deaden the imagination rather than inspire it, I sit down on the firm sofa and indicate that Renee should join me. But she is too agitated to sit. I get back to my feet and we both stand.

'Shall we do some introductions?' I interject, before Ms Rodney can continue. My arm is lightly around Renee's shoulder, to calm her down and try to de-escalate the highly tense situation.

Renee resists my efforts to placate. 'I know you have other children to protect,' she leaps in. 'I know that, but Alex needs protection too.' She spits it out, her arms waving in the air to underscore her point.

'Our policy on offensive weapons and violence is very clear,' Ms Rodney says again, this time with a barely suppressed hiss. 'We can't possibly have Alex in school after fighting and then bringing in a knife. It's simply not safe.'

She takes out her phone and appears to text someone, then returns to the task of making a case for why Alex needs to be excluded. Policy. Safeguarding. An example. She's going through the motions; this is a speech she has given before.

A young man dressed in sports gear comes into the room without knocking. His lean body is preceded by his smartphone. He greets me and Renee with a simple nod, then shows us an image of a knife on his phone. It's displayed on a school desk, a ruler recording its length. The sharpness of its edges are as alarming as the context. If it's intended as a shock tactic, it works.

'This shows you the size of the knife that Alex brought to school. And it shows why it's simply not possible to have him in our school,' Ms Rodney repeats, this time with her words grounded in photographic evidence. 'The police took the knife away as evidence, as I said in my call to your mother. This is now a police case, and we are excluding Alex from our school.'

The fight has gone out of Renee. She sits down abruptly, deflated. Ms Rodney waits.

Eventually, Renee looks up from her lap. 'I am as shocked as you are, Ms Rodney,' she says slowly. 'But please can we find another way around this? What about the boy who fought Alex outside the school gates? Does he get punished?'

I can hear the desperation in her voice, and, as she starts to cry, I realize there's nothing I can do but sit down next to her and offer her some comfort. She curls into me, her head resting under my chin.

When she speaks again, it is into my neck and her voice is muffled: 'Please don't exclude Alex. I know what those PRUs are like. Please don't,' she says through the tears. 'He won't be able to cope in them schools.'

And then, without warning, the fighter in her resurfaces and she sits up to face Ms Rodney. She's not finished yet, it seems.

'Do you know how many Black boys are excluded from school? Do you know how many of them end up in gangs because they are excluded from school?' she shouts. 'A Black boy was stabbed outside a PRU in Woolwich a few months ago. Do you know what this means for Alex?'

But Ms Rodney does not bend. I can't help but wonder how many exclusions she has presided over and if the frequency of the process has inured her to its brutality.

'We have already referred Alex to a Pupil Referral Unit,' Ms Rodney says. 'A reasonably good one, in Barnet. He will be able to continue his education there. They are experienced in working with children with autism and behavioural difficulties.' She seems to think this bald statement will put Renee's mind at rest.

'Well, ain't that the point, though?' Renee persists. 'He has autism and struggles with change, struggles with his emotions. The school – *this* school – should be able to manage that and not exclude him.' Renee sits back, disgusted.

'Ms Rodney, is there anything at all that can be done to reverse this decision?' I ask, finally finding a moment to interject, though I know full well it's unlikely to make any difference. 'In our experience, children who are excluded from school, especially those with learning and adjustment difficulties, can do well in PRUs, but some of them struggle significantly and are vulnerable to being recruited by gangs.'

In 1995, the entire nation was stunned when a teenager stabbed to death a headmaster who was trying to quash a fight outside the gates of his own school in north-west London. Many expected a decline in knife crime after that, but, on the contrary, knife crime by young people, and especially in and around schools, increased. Many parents went to great lengths to try to get their children into schools that were safer, with some opting to move boroughs, postcodes or even towns to secure a place in what they considered to be the best school, with faith and drama schools particularly sought after for their values-based approach to education and the structure they were able to provide.

But here we are again. Ofsted, the government body that inspects schools, has long been concerned about the rise in knife crime in and around schools in the UK, with a general consensus that schools alone cannot tackle violence in education, that a multi-agency approach is needed. Ms Rodney, however, isn't interested in working with us.

'Bringing a knife into school can be considered to be gang activity,' she replies, sternly. She doesn't want gangs forming in her school, but she seems quite happy for them to form elsewhere.

'Before this love-letter thing, Alex was fine in this school...' Renee starts again.

The young man who showed us the image of the knife raises an eyebrow at Ms Rodney as if to say, *This conversation has reached a conclusion. It's time to move on.*

Ms Rodney straightens to her full height and doubles down on her brusque, businesslike manner. 'I am really sorry that it has come to this,' she says dismissively. 'We wish Alex well. He should do well in the PRU, if he adjusts his behaviour.' She smoothly guides us towards the door.

Back in the waiting room, Renee and I sit for a while on the tired sofa. The question for everyone who cares about Alex is, 'Now what?' My mind starts to race, trying to think how I can help to improve his likely poor prognosis. Chattering by my side, Renee is full of ideas, more determined than ever to find a solution for her brother that will support his education, without further compromising his safety. But options for boys like Alex are scarce. I have rarely felt so utterly defeated.

*

What we know so far is that Alex has already been charged by the police for carrying a knife and that he is likely to be given a Youth Offending Team order, typically known as YOT order, which will require him to report regularly to a Youth Offenders Centre. This is Alex's first offence. He is fifteen years old and, because of his age, things are not as bad as they perhaps could be. As yet, his court date has not been set, and I realize that it would be wise to use this window of opportunity – the calm before the storm – to make some progress with my nursing interventions with Alex and the family.

Emotions typically run high in families affected by the systems and structures that they can't help but feel are working against them rather than for them – education, the law, healthcare, social services. Parents whose children are excluded are prone to extreme stress, which can affect their ability to make rational decisions. Anger is common, and it manifests in many different ways. There is a lot of anger in Alex's family. It seems that each family member is trying to cope in their own way and it's pulling them apart rather than bringing them together.

The families that I work with whose children have been involved in stabbings, fighting and bullying are prone to poor physical and mental health, especially where the violence or trauma remains unresolved. My job is to give parents and young people a psychological safe space to express themselves, a space that's rarely afforded to them elsewhere. I need to know about their emotions and how they're responding to internal threat. When they find themselves in a difficult situation, do they feel able to reach out for help, or are they likely to lose control? Do they feel even more anxious if they hear someone else has been attacked or harmed?

Alongside my interventions – the questions I'll ask, in the time given – Miles is tasked with prepping Alex for his court appearance. He'll attend court with Alex and help him to manage his YOT appointments. He'll ensure that Alex gets up on time, dresses appropriately and is versed in the correct etiquette. His demeanour and his language will help to persuade the courts that he is of reasonably good character – or, failing that, of a character that can be rehabilitated. Alex is in good hands with Miles, who's experienced in this work. For my part, Miles has asked if I can address Alex's dad's regular smoking of cannabis in the house; this is not good role-modelling for his son. It's a valid point, but lies slightly outside my remit. I've told him that I think I'll get more traction by working on behavioural modification approaches with Alex, which may well then have a ripple effect on the behaviour of his parents.

To make sure it's the right approach, I bring Alex's case to our regular group supervision meeting with Clinton, our experienced systemic therapist, who's able to draw from his experience of working in multi-agency teams. I am looking for ideas on how to enhance my nursing interventions for young people with knife-crime convictions who are also living with autism. Our team is diverse in experience and, as well as having Clinton's thoughts, I always find our youth workers' views incredibly insightful.

'Help him to regulate his anger,' someone suggests.

'Yes – when he goes to the PRU, he'll be stepping into a space that's going to challenge him. He needs your help to manage his emotions,' another colleague agrees.

'He has been done for carrying a knife, which means that, like in prison, he'll be revered by some, and others will be jealous of him. He will likely have new enemies and the PRU will already have gangs operating. He'll have that to deal with, too,' another youth worker adds.

'But if you and his YOT worker work well together, you could reduce his risk of violence,' someone suggests.

'What about his strengths?' another colleague asks.

The input is coming thick and fast. But it's this last point that stops me in my tracks. It's so easy to view everything through the lens of my clients' vulnerability rather than through their positive character traits. And Alex has such a lot to offer. I wonder if Ms Rodney and the other senior staff at the school ever saw his strengths? And, if they had focused on these, could the whole incident have been handled differently? Better?

For me, Alex's strengths clearly lie in his relationship with his sister. Renee has mentioned that she would like to get Alex into modelling, as she is in touch with a number of agencies through her retail role. It seems so unlikely that Alex could go from where he is now to a career in modelling, but it has to be worth exploring. It may be a stretch, but we can't afford to lose hope.

*

I walk from Kentish Town Tube station to the estate which Alex calls home. Renee, I know, will not be there. She is at work. But she has coordinated the meeting, insisting that an afternoon visit is most appropriate, as Alex has been getting up very late since being excluded from school.

Although he has been enrolled at the PRU in north London, Alex hasn't been attending, partly because he has fears about change and partly because he's worried about crossing postcodes as he makes his way there and back. Miles is helping him with this, using safety- and confidence-building measures. However, it does mean that Alex is missing out on some of his education. His mother and father are ill-equipped to supervise schoolwork at home and Renee has far too much on her plate to be able to help. Transitioning from mainstream education to a PRU can be complex, not least for vulnerable young people with neurodivergent needs. The gap created by the transition increases the risk of gang recruitment and gang involvement. In the absence of a formal education, 'social educators' like drug dealers and gang members can step in.

When the front door opens, Alex towers over me. He half smiles and nods a welcome. His outsize headphones are draped over his head, adjusted so that his ears aren't covered. He is polite as he shows me in, but I can tell that he is tired and his mood is low. As I follow him through to the living room, his body language suggests that he's worn down by the circumstances in which he finds himself. My plan today is to try to understand Alex's emotions – ideally, to get to the bottom of what rejection meant to him when he sent that note to Chantel. Ultimately, I'd like to navigate us around to the big question of why he felt the need to carry a knife to feel safe.

'Why are you like this, Alex?' I can hear his mother speaking from the living room before we get there, her Polish accent still strong. She probes him again: 'When I was growing up, there was no fighting, Alex. Why are you like this?'

I have walked into a conversation – more of an argument – about recent events. Despite all the questions, neither of them has any clear answers. Alex's mother pauses in her outburst to greet me. She has a beer in her hand. She too looks worn out.

As I take a seat in a sagging armchair, she says: 'You know, Alex has always been a sensitive child – even when he was a baby, he was sensitive.'

Alex's developmental history is important information. It's key that I understand his upbringing, his strengths and challenges, and this fuller picture will guide me and the team towards how best to support him. We already know that Alex was born in London, and that his mum struggled with alcohol abuse throughout her pregnancy. We know that, despite this rocky start, he had a fairly happy childhood, playful and caring. I have learned that his autism was suspected early on at primary school and was diagnosed, without too much delay, through the local child and adolescent mental-health clinic. We know that Alex has always been sensitive to change and that his emotional responses have at times been disproportionate and dysregulated. Throughout his childhood, his family encouraged him to be open with his emotions, to play to his strengths not his challenges. But, in Alex's adolescent years, which are happening in a world of hyper social-media engagement over which he has little or no control, he has struggled to judge the risks of being too open about how he feels. It's a balance that he needs to achieve, and should be able to with support from our interventions.

Alex seems comfortable enough with his mother talking about his history and sensitivities, but I can see that he is keen to disappear to his bedroom. I ask if I can speak to him after speaking to his mum, and he agrees.

Alone now, Agnieszka – or Aggy, as she prefers to be called – is more visibly anxious. I hadn't realized that she was wearing a mask for Alex's sake, that the anger was covering her fears. She is worried about Alex being excluded from school, worried about the upcoming court case; both events are weighing heavily on her. Aggy, I learn, works as a healthcare assistant in a nursing home in West London. She's well aware that, given how busy she is, it's Renee who has stepped up to offer the protection and parenting that Alex needs.

Talking with her, it's clear that Aggy's moral compass is firmly anchored to her upbringing – things were very different when and where she grew up, in Poland. Many of my clients' parents who are not originally from the UK find it difficult to reconcile how London can be so violent, when often they moved here in search of safety. I have seen this particularly with parents coming from war-torn environments such as Iraq, Somalia, the Baltic states, the Democratic Republic of Congo, Sudan, Colombia and Syria. There has been little or no research joining the dots between prior exposure to violence and how it informs future violence. Indeed, it would be difficult to conduct such research, given the highly charged politics of immigration and cultural assimilation in the UK and in the Global North more generally.

The circumstances in which Aggy moved from Poland to London are not known to me, neither are the circumstances that brought Alex's dad, Blake, from Dominica to London. It appears that both parents have done their best to raise their children here, but when faced with difficulties they haven't known what to do. They're not alone in being unable to comprehend how their child has been excluded from school – genuinely believing that it's the kind of thing that only happens to other people's children. And, like many people in society, they're struggling to understand how and why some children who are excluded from school end up involved in criminality.

The Office of the Mayor of London has long recognized the link between school exclusion and criminality, and in 2018 reported that London schools had seen a 26 per cent increase in exclusion rates, with research showing that children who are excluded from mainstream education are more likely to be drawn into crime. The report emphasized that children referred to alternative provision, essentially non-mainstream education, are likely to remain there until they finish their GCSEs. It's not a temporary measure, a short, sharp corrective. It is a 'life sentence'. Often presenting at the outset with complex needs such as poor mental health or unstable home environments, these excluded children are made all the more vulnerable.

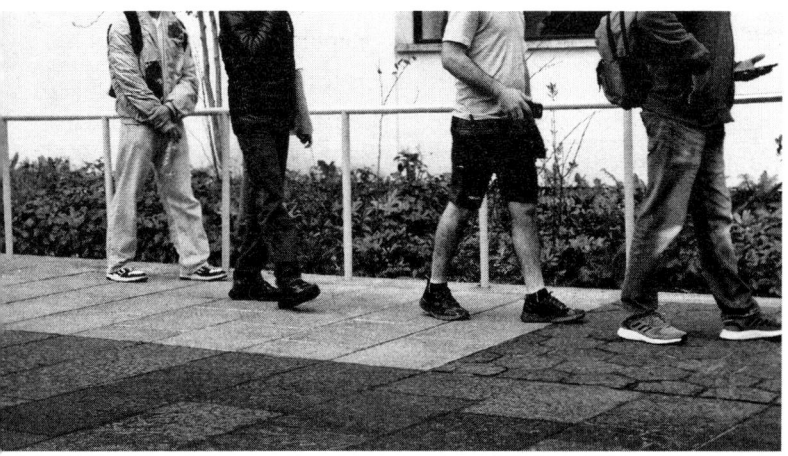

In 2021, researchers Jasmina Arnez and Rachel Condry coined the term 'school to prison pipeline' in their study 'Criminological perspective on school exclusion and youth offending', which considered the vulnerability and exploitation of marginalized children who were excluded from mainstream education. Government data on school exclusion and ethnicity indicates that children from white Gypsy, Roma and Irish Traveller heritage have the highest exclusion rates, with children from Chinese and Indian heritage having the lowest rates of exclusion. Black Caribbean pupils have nearly four times the average exclusion rate. Behind those numbers are real lives, children like Alex who are placed into alternative education programmes that are harmful to their safety and which only increase their future likelihood of carrying a knife. It begs the question, then, what is it that mainstream education offers that Pupil Referral Units do not?

My colleagues and I were often taken a back by the differences. We would compare the two based on our observations of working in both spaces with young people with complex educational needs, who are also frequently neurodivergent. Our conclusion was that while PRUs are committed to supporting their young people through their education they tend to have a higher turnover of staff, which inevitably has an effect on emotional connections being formed and, ultimately, on how safe children feel at school. We could see that PRUs can struggle to find the structure and consistency that mainstream education typically offers.

Within the four walls of Aggy's council-estate home, I let her talk about her feelings of frustration. She reaches for a cigarette with trembling hands and positions herself by the open window to blow smoke outside.

'This must be difficult for you,' I say, validating her feelings.

She drags on the cigarette as if her life depends on it. Then, the tears begin.

I give her space, allowing the silence.

'Will Alex be OK in that new school?' she asks me. 'I hear bad things, very bad things.'

I'd like to be able to reassure her that Alex will be fine at the PRU. I wish I could say that her son will be safe from harm, that he won't be at risk of attack from others, that he will not be lured into more trouble. But I can't. I don't know how Alex will cope. What I can do is ask her about her mood and feelings, and she opens up about how difficult she's finding it to see anything positive in life with everything that's going on. She feels lonely, despite having family around, and cries at night. She blames herself for being emotionally absent because of having to work to keep the family going.

Finding some positivity to cling to, I remind Aggy that the events of the last few weeks are an opportunity to turn things around for Alex and that he needs her love and emotional support to see him through this.

She takes a deep drag on her cigarette and breathes out a sigh of smoke. I sense that she is at least relieved to have been able to talk about it all.

Aggy leaves the lounge, swapping places with Alex. He sits on the sofa, his headphones removed fully now, his head hanging in his hands, his fingers worrying through his short dark hair.

'How are you, Alex?'

He slowly raises his head and looks at me.

'It has been a whirlwind few days,' I acknowledge.

'It's crazy, innit,' he says, with a deep sigh. 'When I wrote that Snapchat message to the girl, I never thought it would come to this.'

Alex, I'm glad to see, is keen to open up.

'The message wasn't even that serious,' he adds, in what may be an attempt to protect his pride. 'The fight was just him jumping on me. Over a girl?' He sounds angry. 'So, I fight him back, innit.'

He pauses. Judging from the fluency with which he's speaking, it's clear he has reflected on what happened, and that is a good thing. As he speaks, I wonder if his anger is self-directed. It's important for me to be clear on this because I do not want Alex to self-harm. So far, at least, there is no indication of this risk. He's not berating himself. I let him vent some more.

'And the knife, that wasn't even that serious. I just carried it, innit,' he continues. 'Now, they're trying to make out like it was all about the knife.'

I don't take for granted the trust he's affording me. Without being aware of quite how vulnerable he is, Alex is looking to me, to our team and to his sister Renee for support. And I'm more keen than ever to support him. My presence in his home is providing a safe space for him to be honest about his feelings. There's no need for artifice here. There's no need to save face. My job is to seek to understand the context of what has happened, never judging or diminishing what someone has been through.

Alex's neurodiverse needs were known to Ms Rodney and her school, and the school will have shared this information with the PRU. But, although the information is known, the truth is that neither institution may understand how Alex experiences the world. Adolescents with autism often struggle to find appropriate responses to the threats they face and, in the absence of structure and emotional security, will reach for that which they perceive to be safe. For Alex, his safety net was a knife. I'm pleased that he has brought up the issue himself. It gives me leeway to discuss it with him. I lean in.

Alex tells me that he brought the knife into school because he feared for his life. He has been in school fights before and experience has taught him that, after a fight is broken up by a member of staff, the other boy will want to fight him again. It is not finished. He planned to threaten the boy with the knife – or, for that matter, anyone else who wanted to fight him. Just a threat. Nothing more, he tells me. In his naivety, he is still unable to see the risk the knife posed to him and everyone around him.

'What would *you* have done, bruv?' Alex asks me, in his innocence.

He is seeking perspective and perhaps considering alternative ways of responding to threats. This is progress. It's now possible to explore how Alex can identify potential threats and how he can manage them. It's work that will require several sessions, but, as with all the young people I look after who are highly exposed to violence, I have to maximize every contact with them as it may well be the last. They might reject my input at any time.

Alex is worried about changing schools, and I am just as anxious about how he will adjust. Still, even in the foothills of this work with Alex, I feel that we are embarking on a journey of heightened self-awareness. Alex is at a junction. He has an opportunity to turn things around, but, if he doesn't seize it, he is likely to take another wrong turn. I am hoping that Alex, who appears willing, won't let that happen.

'How are you coping with it all, Alex?' I ask him.

He pauses, takes a deep breath and says, 'Some days are good, some days I am just sad. Sometimes I smoke my dad's weed – he always has some in the house.'

I am only a little surprised. The young people I work with often use cannabis to cope with stress. But the combination of cannabis use, neurodivergence, anger, violence and poor emotional attachments raises the bar in terms of risk.

All specialist mental-health nurses are highly trained in clinical ethics; we nurse patients who have committed some of the most heinous crimes, and we view them as patients, not as criminals. My compassion for Alex doesn't diminish the offence he has committed – on this, the law must take its course. But I know that at the intersection of law and mental health lies serious vulnerability, and Alex is treading that line. So, while we pay attention to the risks someone like Alex poses to others, as well as sometimes to themselves, we do not lower our standard of care for them. How we get through this is not just a matter for Alex and his family, but for society.

*

In the weeks that follow, Alex leaves home only to attend his Youth Offending appointments, which are stipulated by the courts and enforced by Camden Council. His progress will be monitored through the YOT programme and they will give some consideration to his autism as well as to his fears about integrating successfully into the new education system. Renee is keeping tabs on his progress too. If Alex misses any of his YOT appointments, he runs the risk of being sent to a Young Offenders Institution, which will make a PRU look like a holiday. Should that happen, my concern is that his mental health will be further compromised.

As the days tick over, Alex appears to be developing some sort of social phobia. I have seen this many times in young people who have been involved in violence and are living in fear of further violence. They retreat into themselves, removing themselves from the world. I have nursed young people like Alex who have gone on to develop other conditions associated with social phobia: obesity, anxiety, depression, self-harm and increased substance abuse. I can't let this happen to Alex.

*

In the background, Miles has been doing some conflict-resolution work with the boy Alex fought with. It's a vital part of reducing the risk of retaliation, and involves mediating negotiations between rival groups. Operating alongside other experienced youth workers, and with the involvement of schools, it's a process that's about opening a dialogue and restoring trust in the school and in law enforcement. It's about educating young people and their communities on the value of fostering peace. Sometimes, local councillors are involved too.

Many of our conflict-resolution programmes have their roots in America, where they have been used, with varying degrees of success, in gang-affected neighbourhoods experiencing high mortality rates and trauma – much higher than here in the UK. But London and other cities in the UK need this work to be done too, given the rate at which we are losing young people to knife crime.

These conflict-resolution programmes involve a gathering of elders who are respected by their communities. These are often youth workers and community leaders, many of whom have long exited from gangs or criminality themselves and are now working for reputable charities. The respect is not for their criminal past, but for their ability to use the past to help others. They will often bring with them lower-ranking representatives from both sides of the conflict to meet in a youth club or community hall, with support from the relevant agencies. Parents, teachers and community nurses are invited too. The event is risk-assessed and risk-managed, most often by experienced youth workers.

The shared objective is invariably to slow down or stop the violence altogether. It is here that survivors share their traumatic stories, a parent might stand up and talk about the loss of their child to gang violence, or a teacher might plead with the community to support them with their personal efforts. It's an intervention that Ms Rodney might have benefited from attending, to gain a better sense of the full picture. These conflict-resolution interventions work, but to what degree and for how long depends on the funding and the commitment governments, multi-agencies – social services, the police, healthcare – and communities are prepared to make to save their children's lives.

Miles informs me that Alex has engaged well in the conflict-resolution programme and is keen to place a full stop at the end of this saga. But he remains emotionally fragile and hurt. In search of closure, Alex has written another note to Chantel, which – this time – he shares only with me and Miles.

In the letter, he's once again a teenager in love; there's clearly some residual infatuation with Chantel, but he is also confused by her actions. In his honesty, he tells her how shocked he is about what he feels is a disproportionate turn of events, given all he ever wanted to do was share his feelings for her. He expresses his disappointment in her for sharing his letter with her friends, acknowledging that this act has led to his public shame. He lays bare his feelings, talking openly about how much the gossip which spread like a disease hurt him, how the fight humiliated him, while Chantel and her friends looked on. As if in an act of closure, using words that are really meant for himself, he ends: *But I am alright now.*

It's a poignant note, childlike in its simplicity and all the more powerful for it. And this time, although he's sharing his feelings again, Alex is safe. This time, the note doesn't reach the school bullies, who would have a field day humiliating him for a second time. Writing the note helps with Alex's self-development; the whole process is addressing issues about how adolescents fall in love and how they understand the new and surprisingly powerful emotions they find themselves having for others. What does it mean to feel butterflies in the pit of your stomach for someone? How do young men navigate the issues of consent? What does it mean to be a man, and how do we model masculinity in the absence of good role models?

This is Miles's domain, explored with comprehensive support from the male youth workers who are well versed in working with young men around these issues. My hope is for Alex to come out of this a stronger young man, with a heightened sense of self-awareness, a transformation that will move him away from his current trajectory.

Alex agrees to meet me at his new PRU. After the hiatus, he has been attending the school for two weeks now and has already missed some days. Miles is tasked with encouraging him to attend. He calls on Renee for support, but it seems Renee is still ambivalent about Alex being there and can't be brought on board. She has her eyes on a brighter future for Alex. She is pulling the strings in a different direction, which has left me wondering how Alex is coping with the lack of joined-up thinking from the people around him. If we all want different things for Alex, which way should he jump?

*

The entrance to the PRU is strewn with abandoned Boris bikes, which have been discarded atop a mush of decaying autumn leaves. The school is managed by maintaining a high level of security, and numerous cameras are positioned around the gates and within the school grounds. I pass through a full-body scanning machine and am waved in, approved.

As I enter the reception space, the noise hits me like a force-field. It's much louder than the hubbub I experienced at Alex's previous school, where the underlying tone, though running at a high volume, was one of carefree fun, easy enjoyment. This is different. This feels angry, threatening. I realize that the noise is a combination of pupils' and adults' voices, that the teachers are shouting just as much as their students.

I pull out my nursing badge as ID as I approach the reception desk. My contact is Jonathan, a teaching assistant who is assigned to Alex, given his complex needs. As I wait for Jonathan, I adjust to the environment. This is a place that demands you stay alert. Nearby, a female member of staff seems to be struggling to get a group of pupils into order. She's calling out the adolescents' names, one after the other, according to some kind of register, but none respond. She is effectively talking to herself.

I look more closely at the milling children, eager to catch sight of Alex, but I can't find him in the crowds. All around are young people dressed in casual clothes; there's no uniform here – trying to enforce that would be a complete waste of time. They roam the school corridors – is it break time? – their hands as expressive as their voices.

I take a deep breath. It's not as though I haven't been in this kind of environment before. It reminds me of the many Young Offenders Institutions I have visited around England, with its locked doors, barred windows and blank outdoor spaces that are there to mitigate risk rather than to give the children fresh air. The idea is that there's nowhere to hide.

My anger flares. It's a miserable space for young people who have been outcast from society and I don't know how anyone could possibly flourish here. How can we as a society be content with policy that excludes children from mainstream education only to dump them in places like this and effectively forget about them? It's an environment that's ripe for gang formation, violence, bullying and exploitation. It is the perfect breeding ground for all kinds of vices and criminal activity. Gangs, by their very nature, are about territory, power, violence, drugs and ownership – and I have no doubt they're all thriving here. Alex has already been exposed to most of these simply by being a young man crossing boroughs and postcodes to get to this new school, the journey alone posing risks to his safety. And his arrival here will be interpreted as a threat to other adolescents who are already well established in the codes of conflict and violence, and feel that this is their territory to protect. Even with all that Alex has learned through the conflict-resolution programme, my fear is that it is going to be very difficult for him to come through this experience unscathed.

I feel a light touch on my shoulder and turn.

'You must be the nurse,' a middle-aged man says with a trace of a Scottish accent. He is dressed severely in black and has a thick moustache. His smile is wide and feels far too sunny for the environment in which we're standing.

'Yes, I am. My name's Dorcas.' I shake his outstretched hand.

'I'm Jonathan. I am a teaching assistant here. You've come to see how Alex is getting on,' he says, affirming what we both know. 'We really need a mental-health practitioner in our PRUs, because most of this is mental health, really,' he goes on, with a sweep of his arm towards the milling kids. And then, as if he's speaking to a policymaker, he puts forward a strong case for why mental-health support is needed in these environments.

As he speaks, I nod my head from time to time. He's seemingly unaware that he's preaching to the converted.

'We see a lot of troubled kids here, who don't necessarily fit into the NHS Child and Adolescent Mental Health Services programme – they call it CAMHS. The waiting lists there are ridiculous; kids wait months to see a specialist. And, while they're waiting, their behaviour is just getting worse and worse,' he tells me with passion in his voice. 'Far too many kids are struggling. Some kids self-harm, most of them have anger-management problems, and very few of them can manage their emotions.'

I sense his frustration. A compassionate civil servant tasked with the job of providing education for excluded children, he has little control over policies designed by those above him, yet he's accountable for the children's safety and for their development. His agony is obvious. And yet, throughout, the smile stays on his face.

We're walking side by side along an empty corridor which is in disrepair. The tired walls are bare and our footsteps echo a little. This place has seen some things, for sure. The windows need replacing, I notice – the wooden frames are rotting and the paintwork is peeling away. I can't help but shake my head at the deplorable conditions in this First World education facility, and Jonathan catches the gesture.

'We really try our best here, but our resources are limited – like everywhere else, I guess,' he tells me, a defeated tone creeping in for the first time.

I give him a consoling smile. 'How is Alex getting on?' I ask, bringing the focus back to where it needs to be.

We stop outside a classroom. Quietly, Jonathan reports that Alex has adjusted fairly well, save for the few days of absenteeism that I'm already aware of. Unexplained absence is common for young people enrolled in a PRU. More positively, Jonathan tells me that Alex has faced a couple of encounters with other students which could easily have escalated, but in both instances he made the smart decision to retreat, emerging as the stronger person.

Jonathan admits that there are a few 'groupings' here at the PRU, and I note that he is hesitant to call them 'gangs'. But, whatever the caution around terminology, I know that the police have been called to the PRU several times in recent weeks due to tensions between two of these 'groups', and I'm pleased that Alex has not been involved. Jonathan thinks this is due to the support that Alex is getting – from his sister, Renee, in particular, as well as Miles and myself. Renee may not be engaging with us, but she's still very present in Alex's life. I'm grateful for that.

Debrief over, Jonathan ducks into the classroom and, moments later, Alex emerges.

It has only been a few weeks since I last saw him, but he seems taller somehow, more confident in himself. He has had some maturing to do, that's for sure. Pleased with what I see, I smile.

'You alright, Miss?' he asks.

Despite all the misgivings I've had about this move, about this school, I'm surprised to find that Alex is in a good place mentally. His head is up, his voice is strong. He is smiling. And, as always, he is open about his thoughts and feelings. Standing in the empty corridor, he's happy to report that he is doing well in school, that he is avoiding conflict, despite there being no shortage of opportunities for it. He tells me he has become much better at assessing potential threats and avoiding students who might lead him into trouble. He is keeping up with his YOT appointments, and fully understands the importance of doing so.

Alex tells me he is smoking much less cannabis, and he recognizes that this is because he is feeling less stressed. Besides, he says, he doesn't want to be caught smoking cannabis, which, on top of possession of a knife, would mean running the risk of a sentence at the Young Offenders Institution. It all feels very positive, and I'm chastened; I had no faith that this was the right thing for Alex, but it appears to be working.

And then he says, 'They can't touch my spirit, Miss.'

My heart lurches. He feels as though he's in prison; he's learned how to protect himself from everyone and everything by turning inwards.

This new kid who's standing in front of me – the one who says yes to adults and accepts their support, who not only recognizes but walks away from volatile situations – is someone he has had to construct, having finally understood what it takes not to fail. Alex is still in there, but he has learned to choose his battles well. And the only battle worth fighting is the one that ensures he finishes his YOT programme and emerges safely out the other side.

As I listen to him, I realize that Alex is the sum of our social nursing interventions, of our pulling together. We have achieved this together. Despite the fears Renee and I had about the Pupil Referral Unit, Alex's short time here has had a positive impact on him. The PRU's primary role is to address his complex needs, and they have achieved this – and more. Jonathan and his team, working hand in hand with the other agencies that have scooped Alex up, have managed to keep him safe. They have contained him and supported him. It's a remarkable achievement for an education facility that struggles with a stigma that even I have bought into. A position which I'm quickly having to rethink.

Alex is a success story playing out right before my eyes, and I can't help but be proud of all the hard work and teamwork that has made this happen.

*

Alex's sixteenth birthday comes and goes. I hear from Miles that, building on her brother's new-found stability, Renee has been busy putting him forward to modelling agencies. She is convinced that her younger brother fits the bill, that his striking features will be of interest to fashion brands. I hope she's right. After all, reaching people from different backgrounds is good for business, and representing our society in advertising campaigns – showing that we can and do and must all live together – is a necessary and positive message.

But even if modelling isn't the way forward for Alex, other opportunities are out there. In recent years, many businesses have recognized their social responsibility regarding equity and greater harmony in our increasingly multicultural society. People of colour, who have long suffered the indignities of structural and systemic racism, are high on the agenda in many sectors. Lots of businesses offer training schemes for young people like Alex, helping them to develop skills that will take them off the streets, expose them to possibilities and give them a chance in life. This is good news. The success of the outcome is proportionate to the collective effort – the multi-agency approach – that is put into supporting young people, and of course the readiness of the young person to engage. This intentional focus on social mobility requires compassion. And it involves risk. But, when it goes well, we all win.

I have to confess, the modelling industry scares me; it's not an industry I'm familiar with, but I have some sense of how exploitative it can be. What I do know is that Renee has her brother's back, no matter what. I trust her judgement; her bond with Alex is unshakeable and I can't see her pushing to engage Alex in anything that is even vaguely detrimental to his safety and development.

Out of the blue, Renee calls me for a catch-up and suggests we meet in a cafe near her workplace in Bond Street. As I push through the doors into the crowded space, where every shopper seems to be seeking sanctuary from the rain, Renee is waiting for me at the far end of the room, a latte in hand.

She waves at me, her eyes bright and wide. Her smooth brown skin glows. She is calm, smiling. This is not a Renee that I've seen before. Something has shifted in her, and I can see pride and hope – and perhaps even happiness – in her eyes.

She tells me that she convinced Alex to do a photo shoot for his portfolio, and that he took a bit of persuading. She pulls out a Perspex sleeve of photos and, after a quick wipe with a napkin, spreads them on the table between us.

Alex is dressed in various items of street gear, in different poses, sometimes looking directly into the camera and sometimes looking away. He looks good. Renee tells me about the young professional photographer who was fussing around Alex, directing him to move his body this way and that, and the make-up artist who was on hand to ensure he was looking his best. The photos have been taken around the backstreets of Shoreditch and Islington, the backdrop of the city's graffiti bringing urban

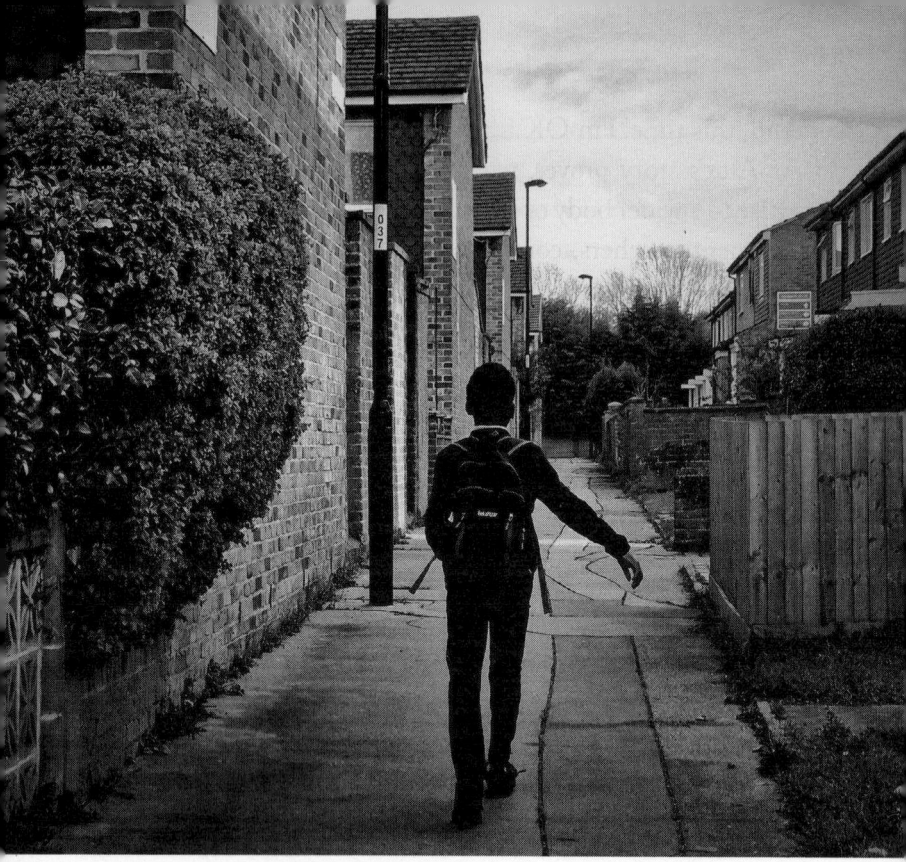

grit but also an unexpected and vibrant glamour. They take my mind back to the waiting room at Alex's school, where all this began, and the education system which almost wrote him off.

Despite the smiles, Renee and I both know that, even though the future looks bright, Alex is still at risk. While his schooling is under control, the uncertainty of this new path could compromise his mental health. Miles, on top of things as always, has pulled in Marvin, a youth worker who has been through the streets himself, to support Alex during this transition into adult life and the working world. And, as a new team around Alex picks up the baton, it's time for me to reduce my contact.

And, this time, I'm OK with that.

As Alex's story proves, when the nursing role contributes expertise to a wider body of multi-agencies – social workers, law enforcement, teachers, community leaders and young people themselves – so much is possible.

Acknowledgements

Over the course of my career, I have nursed people from some of the most vulnerable communities in our society, many of whom have been affected by gangs and knife crime, extremism, FGM, human trafficking, modern slavery, trauma and mental illness. I am deeply grateful to every patient I have looked after. Their vulnerability has pushed my nursing and cultural competency skills, as well as my innovation, to greater heights. Because of them, I will never tire in my quest for a more equal world.

I am deeply grateful to literary agents Martin Redfern, Diane Banks and Matt Cole at Northbank Talent Management, who were able to see this book before I could even imagine it. I owe my deepest gratitude to my editor Andrea Henry for the diligence and care that she has provided, working through draft after draft with thoroughness and deep compassion. To the entire team at Picador – particularly Siobhan Slattery, Elle Gibbons, Kate Tolley, Penelope Price and Tiana-Jane Dunlop – thank you for your support.

I have worked with some of our finest healthcare professionals, many of whom go beyond the call of duty to ensure the highest quality of patient care. The list would be endless if I mentioned everyone, but I would like to single out consultant psychiatrist Dr Maddeline Meile and Million Moyo for affording me the space to grow professionally and personally. They helped me to sharpen my clinical skills, which I then took to the field as I nursed young people through a complex landscape. Their clinical and managerial support have made all the difference. I am immensely grateful.

I am also grateful to the Mary Seacole Foundation as well as the Florence Nightingale Foundation for affording me the grants that made this work possible. My deepest gratitude goes to the Society of Authors for awarding me an Authors' Foundation grant, which allowed me to step back from the frontline and focus on the book.

I am indebted to Dr Tami Kramer and Matt Watson and the entire multi-agency team for embracing me and for supporting the innovation that I brought to my nursing role. I am in awe of the work that you do. This book seeks to honour your efforts to protect vulnerable young people and their families in our city.

I have taken much care in writing about the role of faith and spirituality in safeguarding young people. To ensure that I haven't made any glaring errors, I leaned on the expertise of Dr Mariam Akinpeju Adebayo, Fadzayi Nyirende and Dr Rhoda Molife. I thank them for their measured guidance as I navigated these complex social and cultural landscapes.

In the field of global health, I'd like to pay tribute to all the diaspora workers who are busy on the NHS frontline, bringing innovation from their home countries. They are often invisible and unvalidated. Thank you to Professors Vikram Patel, Dixon Chibanda and Melanie Abas, Dr Nicki Thorogood, and Dr Zed Sibanda for supporting my hunger to contribute to the field of global mental health. To Ben Simms at Global Health Partnerships for years of mentoring and friendship, and for your tireless advocacy for the diaspora. My gratitude to Lord Nigel Crisp for supporting nurses in global health and to Professor Dame E. J. Milner-Gulland for your mentorship in the field of conservation, climate change, youth engagement and safeguarding vulnerable communities.

Over the past few years, I've needed to juggle many roles – frontline nursing, mothering and, for the first time, being a writer. In search of balance, I have often turned to my greatest mentors, Professor Peter Carter, Dr Titilola Banjoko, Ade Adeyemi MBE, Dr Felicia Kwaku OBE, Dr Martin Deahl and Wendy Irwin. This book has been made possible because of their selfless support. I thank you.

In the true African sense, I am a child of great ancestors. While writing this book, I often returned to those who came before us for ancient wisdom, clarity and a deeper sense of compassion. The seeds of storytelling that were planted deep in the rural lands of Zimbabwe and fostered by conversations around crackling fireplaces remind us of the power of the collective, of communities. These values of ubuntu have allowed me to survive my migratory journey, working as a hospital cleaner, training as a nurse, and have subsequently supported the writing of this book.

I am very grateful for the grounding given to me by my parents Julia and Christopher Gwata, who were fierce advocates for equality in their own ways. I thank my sister Ivy Tsindika for providing me with the motherly love, shelter, soulful food and space to write and to be. I am grateful to Dr Knox Chitiyo, Professor Diana Jeater, Tarisai Bere, Sauming Pang, Dr Chido Dziva Chikwari and Lara Sonola for their listening ears and for providing me with the space to think and, again, to write.

Notes

INTRODUCTION

1. ***One in five NHS staff***: Dr Navina Evans, Dorcas Gwata et al., 'Experts in Our Midst: Unlocking the global talent within the NHS', Global Health Partnerships, formerly THET: https://www.globalhealthpartnerships.org/our-work/policy-work/experts-in-our-midst/

2. **46,000 children in England are involved in gangs:** The Children's Society, 'County lines and child criminal exploitation': https://www.childrenssociety.org.uk/what-we-do/our-work/child-criminal-exploitation-and-county-lines

1. FUZ: THE COURTROOM

7. ***At least one in three people moving through the justice system***: Professor Amanda Kirby, 'Neurodiversity – A Whole-Child Approach for Youth Justice', HM Inspectorate of Probation, July 2021: https://www.adhdfoundation.org.uk/wp-content/uploads/2022/08/Neurodiversity-AI.pdf

15. **claiming 285 lives that year**: 'Knife Crime: Fatal stabbings at highest level since records began in 1946', BBC News (website), 7 February 2019: https://www.bbc.com/news/uk-47156957

15. **given the prevalence of guns**: Dominic Casciani, 'Reality Check: Has London's murder rate overtaken New York's?', BBC News (website), 4 April 2018: https://www.bbc.com/news/uk-43628494

2. ABDUL: THE ESTATE

29. *Embarrassing or incriminating social media content*: Keir Irwin-Rogers, James Densley, Craig Pinkney, 'Gang Violence and Social Media', in Jane L. Ireland, Carol A. Ireland and Philip Birch (eds), *The Routledge International Handbook of Human Aggression* (Abingdon: Routledge, 2018).

55. **extended family is also helpful**: Apoorva Ghost, 'After Coming Out: Parental acceptance of young lesbian and gay people', *Sociology Compass*, vol. 14, issue 1, January 2020: https://compass.onlinelibrary.wiley.com/doi/abs/10.1111/soc4.12740

3. LORI: THE CAFE

58. *Minoritised women from particular contexts*: Esmée Fairbairn Foundation, University of Warwick and Imkaan, 'Key findings on sexual violence and Black and minoritised women's interactions with the Criminal Justice System (Reclaiming Voice, 2020)', Prison Reform Trust, 2020: https://www.endviolenceagainstwomen.org.uk/wp-content/uploads/Imkaan-Reclaiming-Voice-CJS-briefing-June-2020.pdf

80. **fewer than 3 per cent of rape cases recorded by the police result in someone being charged**: Rape Crisis England and Wales, 'Rape and sexual assault statistics', accessed April 2025: https://rapecrisis.org.uk/get-informed/statistics-sexual-violence/

4. AMIR: THE MOSQUE

84. *When it comes to socio-economic advantage: having a child with autism can also increase the risk of poverty:* Andres Roman-Urrestarazu, Robin van Kessel, Carrie Allison, Fiona E. Matthews, Carol Brayne, Simon Baron-Cohen, 'Association of Race/Ethnicity and Social Disadvantage With Autism Prevalence in 7 Million School Children in England', *JAMA Pediatrics*, vol. 175, issue 6, June 2021.

97. **Adam Watkins, who published his team's work under the title 'Bad Medicine'**: Adam M. Watkins and Chris Melde, 'Bad Medicine: The relationship between gang membership, depression, self-esteem, and suicidal behaviour', *Criminal Justice and Behaviour*, vol. 43, issue 8, 2016, pp. 1107–26.

5. JORDAN: THE CHURCH

115. ***When gang members embrace religion:*** John Leverso, David C. Pyrooz, James Densley et al. (eds), *The Oxford Handbook of Gangs and Society* (New York: OUP USA, 2024), ch. 28.

6. JEVAUN: THE FOOTBALL PITCH

143. ***Approximately 20 per cent of people:*** Tirion Havard, 'Serious Youth Violence: County lines drug dealing and the Government response', House of Commons Library, 4 February 2022.

144. **They do this by exploiting vulnerable and young people:** 'County Lines', Metropolitan Police (website): https://www.met.police.uk/advice/advice-and-information/cl/county-lines/

7. LOUISE: THE CITY

171. ***Studies have found young women being targeted***: Tirion Elizabeth Havard et al., 'Street Gangs and Coercive Control: The gendered exploitation of young women and girls in county lines', *Criminology & Criminal Justice*, vol. 23, issue 3, 2023, pp. 313–19.

8. HANAD: THE A & E DEPARTMENT

196. ***One in three female and one in ten male gang members***: Karen Hughes, Katherine Hardcastle, Clare Perkins, 'The Mental Health Needs of Gang-Affiliated Young People', Public Health England, 20 January 2015, updated 27 January 2020: https://www.gov.uk/government/publications/mental-health-needs-of-gang-affiliated-young-people

9. ZANE: THE HOUSE

224. ***Private school children are being groomed***: Eleanor Busby, 'Private school pupils being groomed by "county lines" drug gangs, report warns', *Independent*, 14 November 2018: https://www.independent.co.uk/news/education/education-news/private-school-pupils-county-lines-drug-gangs-ofsted-children-grooming-a8633216.html

229. **children of Indian or Chinese heritage**: 'Permanent exclusions', UK Government (website), 11 December 2024: https://www.

ethnicity-facts-figures.service.gov.uk/education-skills-and-training/absence-and-exclusions/permanent-exclusions/latest/

238. **young Black boy living on a council estate**: Research from 2021 indicates that Black and Asian people are more likely to be stopped and searched than their white counterparts. Lara Vomfell and Neil Stewart, 'Officer bias, over-patrolling and ethnic disparities in stop and search', *Nature Human Behaviour*, vol. 5, 18 January 2021, pp. 566–75: https://www.nature.com/articles/s41562-020-01029-w

10. ALEX: THE SCHOOL

255. *Too many children, including some as young as eleven*: Ofsted, Care Quality Commission, HM Inspectorate of Constabulary and Fire & Rescue Services, and His Majesty's Inspectorate of Probation, 'Multi-agency responses to serious youth violence: working together to support and protect children', 20 November 2024: https://hmicfrs.justiceinspectorates.gov.uk/publications/multi-agency-responses-to-serious-youth-violence

269. **It is a 'life sentence'**: 'Bring down school exclusions, bring down violence', Mayor of London/London Assembly (website), https://www.london.gov.uk/programmes-strategies/violence-reduction-unit-vru/bring-down-school-exclusions-bring-down-violence

269. **the vulnerability and exploitation of marginalized children**: Jasmina Arnez and Rachel Condry, 'Criminological perspectives on school exclusion and youth offending', *Emotional and Behavioural Difficulties*, vol. 26, issue 1, 10 April 2021, pp. 87–100: https://www.tandfonline.com/doi/abs/10.1080/13632752.2021.1905233

269. **Government data on school exclusion and ethnicity**: 'Permanent exclusions', UK Government (website), 11 December 2024: https://www.ethnicity-facts-figures.service.gov.uk/education-skills-and-training/absence-and-exclusions/permanent-exclusions/latest/

270. **a feeling of transience**: Hannah Stancliffe, 'Comparing PRUs With Mainstream Secondary Education System', York St John University blog, 16 June 2021: https://blog.yorksj.ac.uk/alternativeeducationsyorksj/2021/06/16/comparing-prus-with-mainstream-secondary-education-system/

A Note on the Photography

Chanel Pinnock was born and lives in south London. She is interested in art in all its different forms, and particularly enjoys working with her hands. Being creative is not just a passion, it is how she communicates who she is on the inside to the outside world. She works in collaboration with the Inside Out Clothing Project, which is the UK's first sustainable fashion brand designed by first-time ex-offenders. More than a brand, it's a movement redefining opportunity, second chances and the power of creativity. The project empowers young adults (eighteen- to thirty-five-year-olds) with the skills, mentorship and industry connections to rebuild their futures through fashion, digital literacy and entrepreneurship. From pop-up shops to an online store and high-profile collaborations – including partnerships with the NFL and global fashion leaders – the Inside Out Clothing Project provides a platform for untapped talent to thrive. Through training programmes, work experience and prison outreach, it equips participants with the tools to succeed, while reshaping societal perceptions. It is more than fashion. It's freedom through fashion, transformation through design, and resilience through creativity – one bold idea at a time.

For more information see https://www.insideoutpjt.com

About the Author

Dorcas Gwata is an award-winning nurse specializing in mental health, a Global Mental Health consultant and an adviser at Global Health Partnerships. She is an accident-and-emergency specialist nurse and has worked within multi-agency teams in the UK and with global-health partnerships focusing on Africa and Asia. Her work with young people and families affected by gang culture in London grew out of innovative evidence-based research in low-income countries extrapolated to high-income countries, improving mental-health outcomes in vulnerable groups while addressing health inequalities in the UK. *The Street Clinic* is her first book.